SUBSTANTIAL
RELATIONS

SUBSTANTIAL RELATIONS

Making Global Reproductive Medicine
in Postcolonial India

Sandra Bärnreuther

CORNELL UNIVERSITY PRESS   ITHACA AND LONDON

Thanks to generous funding from the Swiss National Science Foundation, the ebook editions of this book are available as open access volumes through the Cornell Open initiative.

First published 2021 by Cornell University Press

ISBN 978-1-5017-5819-5 (hardcover)
ISBN 978-1-5017-5820-1 (pdf)
ISBN 978-1-5017-5821-8 (epub)

Library of Congress Control Number: 2021944996

DOI: https://doi.org/10.7298/0rf-ds33

Chapter 1 was first published in *Zeitschrift für Ethnologie* 143:41–60 under the title "From Urine in India to Ampoules in Europe: The Relational Infrastructure of Human Chorionic Gonadotropin." An earlier version of chapter 2 appeared in the article "Innovations 'Out of Place': Controversies over IVF Beginnings in India between 1978 and 2005," *Medical Anthropology* 35 (1): 73–89, DOI: 10.1080/01459740.2015.1094066, https://www.tandfonline.com/.

Für Cilli und Hans

Contents

Acknowledgments

Research always constitutes a collaborative endeavor. Nevertheless, I could not have imagined the countless people who would help along the way when I started this project more than ten years ago. I am deeply grateful to all research partners who patiently and generously shared their knowledge and lives with me. I hope this book does justice to the diverse experiences connected to reproductive medicine in India.

Although I cannot possibly mention all interlocutors, and I can only use pseudonyms, I start with the people who taught me everything I know about IVF in India. First of all, I am much obliged to the many IVF patients in Delhi for their openness and cordiality and for allowing me to be present during these private and often trying moments of their lives. I also thank the doctors and clinical staff who kindly accommodated me in their busy schedules. Special thanks go to the physician I call Dr. Nishika, who permitted me to observe clinical life in her private hospital over several months, as well as the junior doctors, nurses, and staff working there. I am also deeply indebted to the clinicians, nurses, and staff of one of Delhi's public IVF centers, who put up with a curious observer and warmly welcomed me to the team. Furthermore, I am immensely grateful to the many people in Kolkata, Mumbai, and Delhi who generously shared their experiences and views on the history of IVF in India. Particularly Sunit Mukherjee was a huge source of support. One of the most humble and kind-hearted persons, he continued to inspire me since we first met in 2012. Unfortunately, he passed away in Kolkata on January 4, 2020. He will be missed and remembered. I also owe thanks to the staff working for various archives who were incredibly supportive in providing material, as well as Arpita Gosh, who helped with Bengali translations.

This book started at the Cluster of Excellence "Asia and Europe in a Global Context" and the South Asia Institute at the University of Heidelberg. The groundwork was set during research in Delhi, Kolkata, and Mumbai between 2010 and 2014. During most of my stays in Delhi, I was affiliated with Jawaharlal Nehru University and accommodated in a student hostel. I greatly profited from engaging conversations with scholars and students, particularly at the Centre for the Study of Social Systems and the Centre of Social Medicine and Community Health. I am grateful to Harish Naraindas, who facilitated my stay, for his critical mind and for always challenging assumptions. I also thank Burton Cleetus, Tulsi

Patel, Mohan Rao, Sunita Reddy, and Sujata V. for important insights and advice. Life at JNU would not have been the same without some incredibly welcoming friends. Although *dosti me no sorry no thank you*, I would like to mention Sneha Banerjee, Ruchira Bhattacharya, Padma Dolma, Samina Khan, Vivek Kumar, and Nidhi Mittal, who always offered critical inputs, helpful suggestions, and much-needed humor during walks and *dhaba* chats. Heartfelt thanks also go to the many other friends in Delhi and Kolkata who have accompanied me through-out these years—most notably, Chhandak Pradhan, whose calmness keeps me grounded and whose positivity makes my life brighter every day.

During the writing process, I found a first intellectual home at the South Asia Institute in Heidelberg. I am greatly indebted to Eva Ambos, Christoph Berg-mann, Cristoph Cyranski, Sarah Ewald, Aditya Ghosh, Marion Herz, Verena La Mela, Sinjini Mukherjee, Karin Polit, Laurent Pordié, Paul Roden, Bo Sax, Nike-Ann Schröder, Christian Strümpell, and Anna-Lena Wolf for the always-helpful conversations and their astute feedback on early drafts. I also thank the members of the doctoral colloquium at the Department of Social and Cultural Anthropol-ogy, who contributed considerably to shaping some of the arguments I make in this book. My second intellectual home was the Department of Social and Cul-tural Anthropology at the University of Zurich, where I also conducted the bulk of historical research for this book. I thank Johannes Quack for his extraordinary mentorship and support. Olivia Killias, Esther Leemann, Juliane Neuhaus, and Irina Wenk helped me more than they can imagine. Without their constructive critique, encouragement, and solidarity this book would not have seen the light of day. Huge thanks also go to Sneha Banerjee, Nolwenn Bühler, Stefan Leins, Francesca Rickli, and Emanuel Schäublin, who read different chapters and pro-vided valuable feedback.

This manuscript also profited from periods of time that I spent at various other academic institutions as well as from engagements with scholars all over the world. During my time as a Fulbright fellow at New York University, Emily Martin and Rayna Rapp were local advisers and provided much valued intellec-tual inspiration. I am also immensely grateful to Nayantara S. Appleton, David Arnold, Dwai Banerjee, Supurna Banerjee, Aditya Bharadwaj, Janet Carsten, Jacob Copeman, Risa Cromer, Anirban Das, Daisy Deomampo, Tiana B. Hayden, Gabriela Hertig, Larisa Jasarevic, Roger Jeffery, Heidi Kaspar, Janina Kehr, Naya-nika Mathur, Townsend Middleton, Sebastian Mohr, Projit B. Mukharji, Vijay-anka Nair, Tamar Novick, Luisa Piart, Celia Roberts, Mihir Sharma, Christy Spackman, Sayantani Sur, and Miriam Wenner for having been encouraging conversation partners at different points of time during this project.

In light of busy schedules and urgent deadlines, reviewing a book-length manuscript seems like a burdensome task. I am therefore incredibly thankful to the anonymous reviewers for their time and effort. Their critical comments and valuable suggestions were highly appreciated. Thanks are also due to the wonderful team at Cornell University Press, particularly Clare Kirkpatrick Jones, Jim Lance, and Susan Specter, who supported this project from the beginning and managed all the background work that it takes to finally see a book in print.

I acknowledge the institutional support of the Cluster of Excellence "Asia and Europe in a Global Context" at the University of Heidelberg, which provided three years of funding for the initial research. A two-year research grant by the Indo-Swiss Joint Research Programme in the Social Sciences jointly funded by the Indian Council for Social Science Research and the Swiss State Secretariat for Education, Research and Innovation allowed follow-up visits in Delhi as well as in-depth historical research. During other phases of this project, I profited from a Fulbright fellowship at New York University, two fellowships by the research network "Advances in Research on Globally Accessible Medicine" at the University of Edinburgh and Jawaharlal Nehru University, a research fellowship at the Institute of Advanced Study at Jawaharlal Nehru University, and a CSASP fellowship at the School of Global and Areas Studies, University of Oxford, which was supported by a scientific exchanges grant from the Swiss National Science Foundation (IZSEZ0_183350). I further thank the Swiss National Science Foundation for generously funding the open access publication of this book (10BP12_200196).

Last, and most important, I cannot thank my family, particularly my parents, enough for their love, which has sustained me throughout happy and harsh times. Without their unconditional support this book would not have come to life. It is dedicated to them.

Note on Transliteration

Hindi and Bengali words are italicized and transliterated following rules that are guided by the International Alphabet of Sanskrit Transliteration but adjusted for readability. Personal names, place names, and common concepts (e.g., *karma*) are incorporated into the running text without diacritical signs.

SUBSTANTIAL RELATIONS

Introduction

Colorful balloons adorn the entrance to the Annual Test Tube Baby Get-Together that is organized in an upper-middle-class neighborhood in Kolkata (formerly Calcutta), the capital of the East Indian state of West Bengal, by an in vitro fertilization (IVF) hospital. Pink and white tents await the guests in the park opposite the hospital. It is still early, yet an inflatable castle and a carousel are already taken over by kids. Young men wearing the costumes of popular Indian cartoon characters are joking around behind the castle. Heaps of presents have been unloaded from the hospital ambulance and carried into the main tent, which is slowly beginning to fill up. Former infertility patients from different parts of India and socioeconomic backgrounds are invited to attend the get-together with their children. Along with receiving gifts, they will hear speeches, enjoy an entertainment program, and have lunch. But, most important, they have come to meet Dr. Baidyanath Chakraborty.[1]

Dr. Chakraborty is a well-known IVF physician—a "doyen," as he is often called, and an instrumental figure in the making of global reproductive medicine in India. His career has been deeply intertwined with (trans-)national IVF history. He was associated with a company that sourced biological material in Kolkata and exported it to Europe in order to manufacture pharmaceuticals used for IVF. More important, he was a colleague of Dr. Subhas Mukherjee, who has been credited in India as the creator of the country's first IVF baby in 1978. Later, in the 1980s, Dr. Chakraborty conducted his own IVF experiments in a small clinic, where he converted an adjoining garage into a laboratory. The Annual Test Tube

Baby Get-Together today is organized by his new hospital. "From a cowshed to this institute," is how he summarizes his professional trajectory—a somewhat emblematic success story that aptly conveys the transformation of IVF over the past decades: from an experimental research project conducted by clinicians as a hobby, to a standardized product and profitable industry.

Suddenly, a white car makes its way through the gate to the entrance of the tent. While getting out, Dr. Chakraborty is immediately surrounded by former patients who prostrate before him, touch his feet, or put their children into his arms in order to receive blessings and take photographs. Many IVF patients in India—particularly after they become pregnant—state that their doctors are like "god" to them. The doctors succeeded in giving them what most had tried to attain for years: offspring. Celebrations like the Test Tube Baby Get-Together that are organized by many hospitals all over India parade this success, while conveniently concealing from public gaze the many patients whose procedures have failed.

The tent has filled up, and people are standing to greet Dr. Chakraborty. After he has braved the crowds, the speeches on stage start. Dr. Chakraborty welcomes his guests with introductory remarks. Infertility, he says, is a curse for families. But it is a condition that can be cured through reproductive medicine—as the living proof around him attests. This publicly conveyed optimism is often overshadowed by uncertainty in daily clinical practice. After all, failure rates for IVF cycles worldwide are as high as 65 percent, according to the European Society for Human Reproduction. Dr. Chakraborty goes on to emphasize that the performance of IVF babies in professional and social life is excellent—a fact that is visualized by a talent show, during which IVF children dance, sing, recite poems, and play musical instruments. Dr. Chakraborty's comments are certainly reassuring in a cultural setting where IVF is sometimes considered to be an "unnatural" procedure and often kept secret. In this way, the Test Tube Baby Get-Together as a public spectacle not only advertises IVF as a medical intervention but also contributes to its normalization in India.

After the speeches, guests line up to take photographs with Dr. Chakraborty while a magician and his assistant take over the stage. They dazzle the audience by turning sticks into flowers and pieces of cloth into rows of flags. They transform substances—much like IVF does, which a nurse once jokingly called a "kind of magic." In the clinic and laboratory, bodies designated as infertile are turned into gamete producers, egg cells and sperm are turned into embryos, and donor gametes from "outside" the family are turned into one's "own" offspring.

In this book, I think through substances—materially and metaphorically—to illustrate the making of global reproductive medicine in India.[2] Tracing travels and transformations of substances over space and time, I offer a historical and

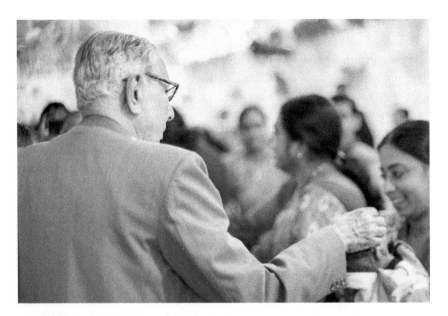

FIGURE 1. Dr. Chakraborty at the Annual Test Tube Baby Get-Together. Photo by Chhandak Pradhan.

ethnographic exploration of the relations generative of and generated by reproductive medicine in India across various scales: from transnational connections between the urban poor in Kolkata and the pharmaceutical industry in Europe to unequal relations between supposed centers and peripheries of knowledge production; from hidden ties between gamete donors and recipients to the minute engagements of medical professionals with gametes and embryos. Substances, I argue, constitute "useful linking figures as ethnographers follow complex, multisited, and multiscalar phenomena" (Shapiro and Kirksey 2017, 481), such as reproductive medicine.

Making Global Reproductive Medicine in India

Since the 1980s, an exciting body of scholarly work on reproductive medicine and assisted reproductive technologies has emerged within the broader disciplinary fields of medical anthropology, science and technology studies, and gender studies.[3] Initially, most scholars focused on reproductive technologies in Euro-America.[4] Since the 2000s, however, many have started to pay attention to their global spread.[5] This has led to various studies of particular locales in the "global

South," which provide fascinating accounts of how reproductive medicine has materialized and is consumed in specific sites.[6] They demonstrate that IVF is practiced in similar and simultaneously different ways in various parts of the world.[7] Along these lines, IVF in India can be described as constituting a "global form" (Ong and Collier 2005; Knecht, Klotz, and Beck 2012) with specific local interpretations and appropriations (Appadurai 1996).

This perspective, however, may at times carry subtle overtones of an implicit dichotomy between centers and peripheries of medical research and practice: while centers, located within the "global North," conduct research and produce knowledge, peripheries only practice medicine and reinterpret technologies. Highlighting India's productive role in shaping global reproductive medicine, in this book I attempt to go beyond aspects of application and adaptation. One salient example is the case of Dr. Subhas Mukherjee. As a physician in Kolkata, he declared himself to have created a "test-tube baby" in 1978, the same year the first IVF baby was born in the United Kingdom. His claim was dismissed at first, as it was perceived to be an "innovation out of place." Starting in the late 1990s, however, his contributions to reproductive medicine have been recognized, at least among medical circles in India. Therefore, a crucial question I ask is not only how global reproductive medicine is being practiced in India today but also how it has been made there over time. By offering a diachronic analysis that emphasizes India's longstanding connections and contributions to this medical field, I attempt to "eschew simplistic binary classifications between Euro-American medical and scientific practice and local epistemologies" (Copeman 2013, 196). This is neither to deny global power asymmetries nor to provide a glorified, nationalistic narrative but to emphasize that "no regional account of the emergence of IVF is ever just an isolated local one. Ultimately they are all world histories involving complex connections across time and space" (Franklin and Inhorn 2016, 4).

In the first part of the book, I trace the genealogy of India's position within global reproductive medicine from the 1960s up to the present day through three critical moments: the sourcing of Indian bodily material for a Dutch pharmaceutical company between the 1960s and 1990s, contestations around the first IVF experiments in the country between the 1970s and 2000s, and the emergence of a transnational IVF sector in India since the late 1980s. Following the sometimes smooth but oftentimes turbulent travels of bodily material, knowledge claims, medical supplies, and financial investments, I highlight India's shifting role throughout its postcolonial history: from a provider of raw material to a producer of knowledge and, subsequently, a thriving medical market that, by now, attracts patients from all over the world.

After analyzing these formations historically, in the second part of the book I examine IVF's contemporary making in fine-grained ethnographic detail. Entering the realms of hospitals and laboratories in Delhi, I turn IVF practice itself into an object of inquiry (Kahn 2000).[8] While this book builds on many excellent accounts depicting experiences of infertility and the use of reproductive technologies in India (Bharadwaj 2016; Mulgaonkar 2001; Singh 2017; Widge 2001, 2005), I seek to move beyond patients' (and sometimes doctors') perspectives alone. Foregrounding the "daily grind" (Wahlberg 2018, 13) in hospitals and laboratories, my analysis focuses instead on IVF at work. More specifically, I show how IVF is made to work through a delicate "ontological choreography" (Thompson 2005) of patients, clinicians, embryologists, biological material, pharmaceuticals, technologies, guidelines, protocols, and so on. This choreography, however, is precarious—a reason why experiences of failure, anxiety, and unpredictability are prevalent in IVF hospitals.

The book thus takes a fresh look at reproductive medicine in India: from questions around its present *use* toward an inquiry into its historical and contemporary *making*. Rather than considering reproductive medicine as a stable clinical product to be consumed, I explore it as a phenomenon that has been formed historically and is being shaped through everyday practice.

But how to analyze a complex phenomenon in the making? Scholars have used various notions, such as (reproductive) assemblage (Ong and Collier 2005; Inhorn 2015) or complex (Wahlberg 2018; see also Franklin 2013), to "capture the ways in which particular juridical, medical, social, economic, cultural, and institutional configurations are consolidated over time and in particular places" (Wahlberg 2018, 8). I find it particularly useful to think about global reproductive medicine in India as an "assemblage" that is constantly "shifting, in formation, or at stake" (Ong and Collier 2005, 12). The notion spotlights the various scales that reproductive medicine spans and conjoins: from the past to the present, from the monumental to the microscopic. On a temporal level, reproductive medicine can be described as "composed of con-temporary elements . . . each with its distinctive moment of origin" (Rees 2018, 86). Similar to a car that "is a disparate aggregate of scientific and technical solutions dating from different periods" (Serres and Latour 1995, 45, as cited in Rees 2018, 84), the elements that constitute reproductive medicine emerged at distinct times. IVF, for instance, conjoins research on embryology and animal experiments since the nineteenth century with technologies of the twentieth and twenty-first centuries, such as cryopreservation and EmbryoScopes (A. Clarke 1998). In addition to temporal scales, reproductive medicine also fuses distinct geographical scales. It entails the transnational movement of biologicals, pharmaceuticals, technologies, knowledge, and patients. It depends on global economic regimes, ethical guidelines, national policies, and legal frameworks. It is debated in scientific journals, at international conferences, in local media outlets, but also within the walls of private homes. And it is practiced in hospitals, inside laboratories, and within bodies and cells. Blending temporal and spatial scales, reproductive medicine appears as an intricate phenomenon that requires careful historical *and* ethnographic analysis. My aim therefore is not only to provide a snapshot of a specific temporary stabilization of this assemblage but to trace its "systems of relations" (Wahlberg 2018, 10) over space and time.[9] In order to examine relations that are generative of and generated by global reproductive medicine in India, I use substances as a connecting thread. In short, I analyze the making of global reproductive medicine in postcolonial India through the prism of substances and relations.

Thinking through Substances

The notion of "substance" has proven to be "good to think with" in anthropological scholarship (Carsten 2001, 30). According to Janet Carsten, the term has a wide range of meanings in English, which she reduces to "four broader categories: vital part or essence; separate distinct thing; that which underlies phenomena; and corporeal matter" (2004, 111). It is exactly this multivocality—the consolidation of different dimensions—she argues astutely, that makes the notion productive. Furthermore, in her comparison of distinct uses of the term in anthropological analyses, Carsten detects a "co-optation of substance to express mutability and transformability, the flow of objects of bodily parts between persons, and the capacity to stand for the relations between those persons" (2001, 49). Over the course of this book, I focus on relational aspects of substances and play with the notion of "substantial relations," employing it in several ways: (1) the substantial (i.e., significant) flows vital for the making of reproductive medicine, (2) the relational potential of biological substances, and (3) the relational constitution of biological substances in hospitals and laboratories.

Vital Flows

In the first part of the book, I mainly rely on Carsten's first category when I follow the transnational and multidirectional travels of biological material, knowledge claims, medical supplies, and financial investments as *vital parts* that have animated global reproductive medicine.[10] One could even describe them as reproductive substances in a metaphorical sense—as substances bringing forth reproductive medicine. A hormone derived from the urine of pregnant women in Kolkata, for instance, used to be a prominent component of a pharmaceutical manufactured in the Netherlands that was fundamental for the reproductive industry. This hormone provided by Indian donors and exported to Europe enabled medical interventions for infertility patients all over the world. Conversely, flows of technologies and money from different parts of the world to India have provided the material and financial base for the enormous growth of the country's IVF sector since the 1990s.

An emphasis on flows, however, tends to underexpose the stratified terrains through which substances travel. While the hormone human chorionic gonadotropin (hCG) derived from the urine collected in Kolkata moved rather easily across international borders, slower to follow were knowledge claims, medical supplies, and financial investments. As Marcia Inhorn perceptively points out, "reproflows" are oftentimes "blocked, hindered, or rendered inert" (2015, 26). For example, in the 1970s and 1980s, many technologies, pharmaceuticals, and consumables necessary for IVF were very costly in India because of high import duties. IVF experiments therefore relied on the inventiveness of doctors who assembled machines or smuggled medications and disposables. Yet stratified topologies morph over time: the 1990s and 2000s witnessed the rise of medical distributors in India due to the country's economic reforms, which were a crucial prerequisite for the flourishing of the contemporary IVF industry. In the first part of the book, I attend to these dynamics in postcolonial India and trace the vital flows that have provided the conditions of possibility not only for the country's thriving IVF sector but for global reproductive medicine on a larger level.

Relational Potential of Substances

In the second part of the book, the fourth category of Carsten's typology gains prominence, when I explore contemporary IVF work through the lens of *corporeal matter*. Defined as fertilization in vitro—that is, fertilization outside the body—IVF is largely characterized by the disembodiment of and work with reproductive substances.[11] Tracing the travels and transformations of biologicals within IVF hospitals and laboratories, I examine the various kinds of connections generated: between parents and offspring, donors and recipients, or professionals and biologicals. I am interested in what relations, from the clinical to the commercial, from the epistemic to the ethical, are summoned by substances in daily medical practice.

The relational potential of substances has long constituted a prominent theme in South Asian studies, particularly with regard to personhood, kinship, and caste. Scholars have illustrated how exchanges of "substance-codes" through daily interactions are consequential in that they create forms of relatedness in North India (Marriott 1976, 1990; Marriott and Inden 1977).[12] As these exchanges are supposed to happen in a controlled manner (e.g., within the bounds of specific kinship or caste groups), they are highly regulated and policed. But what happens when such notions of relatedness meet biomedical possibilities of reproductive exchange (e.g., the mobility of biological substances in IVF clinics)?[13] On the one hand, I describe how IVF is experienced as a useful tool to establish substantial relations between parents and their "own" offspring. On the other hand, the seemingly boundless circulation of biologicals within IVF centers also leads to anxieties about mix-ups and boundary transgressions. The moment during my fieldwork when the mother of a patient asked her daughter after the embryo transfer whether she had checked that her own embryos were put back into the uterus aptly conveys the sense of unease with which many people in India approach IVF.

Although much anthropological work "focuses on the uses to which substance has been put in the analysis of kinship" (Carsten 2004, 116), I explore relations forged through substances that go beyond kinship. The hormone hCG, for example, not only connects the urban poor in Kolkata with infertility patients worldwide but also entangles regions in the global South deeply affected by structures of colonial extraction with thriving bioeconomies in the global North. In this case, "relations extend . . . and create interconnections with landscapes, production, and consumption, requiring us to tie the history of technoscience with political economy" (Murphy 2008, 697). The remarkable scholarship on contemporary bioeconomies that has traced global connections through a focus on biological substances is a case in point (e.g., Almeling 2011; Kroløkke 2018; Waldby 2019; Waldby and Mitchell 2006).

It is important to stress that relations generated by substances are of distinct quality: some might be intended, others unwanted; some might be nourishing, others exploitative; some might be intense, others fragile. When offspring are born and patrilineages continued through IVF, relations are often desired. However, in cases in which donor gametes enter the reproductive process, patients usually try to erase what they consider to be inappropriate substantial relations, particularly if sperm or egg donors are of a different religion or caste. They mobilize silence and secrecy in order to be able to acknowledge children conceived through donor gametes as their "own."

Relations may also be defined by their inequality. In many instances, global reproductive medicine is practiced on uneven ground. This becomes obvious from the unremarkable parcels that left the airport in Kolkata by plane almost every week between the 1970s and 1990s, which contained partly purified hCG, the hormone derived from urine donated by pregnant women in Kolkata's outskirts. Their destination was an industrial town in the Netherlands, where a pharmaceutical company purified and processed the product to manufacture hormone preparations. While the final pharmaceutical product was used for fertility interventions in the global North, it was hardly available in India at the time. This is just one example of how reproductive medicine thrives on unequal relations. Scholars working on contemporary surrogacy arrangements in India have provided excellent accounts of similar transnational inequalities with regard to labor (Vora 2013; Pande 2014; Rudrappa 2015) and racial imaginaries (A. Banerjee 2014; Deomampo 2016) that still structure reproductive medicine. Today, inequalities also exist between Indian IVF patients in different kinds of hospitals in Delhi, as is reflected in the stratified ways in which gametes circulate. While in high-cost hospitals a couple's right to ownership over their gametes is emphasized, couples in low-cost hospitals are often expected to generously share substances with others.

Along with quality, the intensity of relations may vary and shift over time. Relations may be generated and maintained or loosened and ruptured. By depicting relations as "preeminently dynamic in nature, as unfolding, ongoing processes rather than as static ties among inert substances" (Emirbayer 1997, 289), I highlight their historicity and fluidity. This becomes apparent in the ways in which patients "flow through the clinic" (Inhorn 2015, 26) in their quest for substantial relations. Rather than a narrative of progress from infertility to completed family, "'negative' temporalities of delay or failure" (Abram and Weszkalnys 2011, 14) were prominent experiences. Many of my interlocutors had a history of convoluted treatment trajectories that included detours, suspension, repetition, and setbacks. These dynamics show how patients' relations to infertility and medical interventions fluctuate with the passage of time.

Relational Constitution of Substances

In a last step, I explore how substances themselves are constituted relationally. In this way, apart from relations between things, "things *as* relations" (Strathern 1995, 19; my emphasis) become the center of analytic attention. How are biological substances—from bodies to gametes to embryos—constituted in clinics and laboratories? What kind of relations shape them and render them valuable for IVF? And how do medical professionals and patients in turn relate to those substances? Examining these questions, I "un-blackbox" (e.g., Latour and Woolgar 1986; Latour 1999) biologicals to showcase the relations through which they become viable and valuable. For example, gametes or embryos become biologically relevant only when they are cultured and sometimes even enhanced in the laboratory; most bodies become medically useful only once they are prepared with hormones; and urine becomes economically productive only after it has been collected and processed. Seen in this light, "things, objects, entities achieve their significance in terms of their relationships" (M'charek 2013, 421; see also Abrahamsson et al. 2015).

This implies that biological substances are never only "life itself." Rebecca Marsland and Ruth Prince's (2012) notion of "life as such" (see also Fassin 2009), in the sense of "life as lived through both a body and a society," is useful here. The living, they suggest, "is a cultural and historical product, and one which may well look different in the varied locations in which we work" (Marsland and Prince 2012, 462; see also Merleau-Ponty 2017). In this sense, "a frozen embryo in Delhi is not the same as a frozen embryo in London or Quito" (Roberts 2012, 4). Embryos may appear as "icons of life" (Morgan 2009), as they often do in pro-life debates in the United States (Cromer 2018), but they may also come to matter in distinct ways. Laboratory practice and clinical work in most IVF hospitals in Delhi reveal a more fluid understanding of embryos in terms of a process of becoming rather than a form of existence

Although biological substances are constituted through specific relations and contexts, they are not completely determined by them. While patients' bodies, for instance, are fashioned within the pharmaceutical regime of IVF, they recursively engage with medical practice. Bodies "respond," as clinicians call it (for the concept of "kicking back," see Barad 1998). Similarly, embryologists engage with gametes and embryos as substances that constantly surprise them. The interference of biologicals with medical interventions becomes apparent in the many moments of failure prevalent in IVF clinics. I therefore show how clinicians and embryologists address unpredictability as a central epistemological and ethical challenge in hospitals and laboratories.

All in all, thinking through substances, whether understood materially or metaphorically, allows us to explore the manifold connections that reproductive medicine relies on and generates on distinct levels. It gives insights into global and historical dynamics without losing sight of the intricacies of contemporary clinical life and intimate bodily experiences. In short, it tracks global reproductive medicine as a complex and shifting assemblage. In the following, I illustrate the specific historical, political, and economic culture that has nourished IVF in India and show the different ways that reproductive medicine, in turn, has fashioned India's postcolonial history.

Culturing IVF

Science and medicine in the subcontinent have long been contested arenas with complex political and economic histories.[14] And reproductive medicine has been right at the center, especially as populations have become crucial targets for state interventions since the nineteenth century (Arnold 1993). The issue of infertility, however, has long remained in the shadows of the rigid population control efforts that mark this history. Even before India's Independence, a subcommittee of the National Planning Committee, founded by the Indian National Congress in 1938, "favoured birth control in the interest of the development of the nation, thus linking individual and family behaviour to national growth" (Rao 2004, 20). In 1952, India became the first country worldwide to launch a family planning program—a target-based approach that cumulated in a system of incentives and the infamous sterilization camps of the 1970s and 1980s (Tarlo 2003; Rao 2004). That India has been at the forefront of infertility research, as the birth of its first IVF baby in 1978 attests, might therefore seem surprising. But medical work on contraception and infertility often cross-fertilized each other.[15] During the 1980s, the Institute of Research in Reproduction in Mumbai ran the first publicly funded IVF program in India with the hope that the project would answer basic questions in the field of reproductive biology. The research program was also justified by the following rationale: if a method could be developed that allowed people who had been sterilized and then lost their children to conceive again, more people might accept permanent family planning procedures (*ICMR Bulletin* 1984, as cited in Mukherjee and Nadimipally 2006, 129; see also Anand Kumar et al. 1988). It was thus only because of its conceptualization as a technology of birth control that IVF practice became possible in India at that time (for China, see Wahlberg 2018, 6). Although IVF has since been normalized as a medical intervention for infertility and is used in urban areas by a wide range of people, questions of whether a country of more than one billion people should utilize public money to support such an expensive procedure as IVF have continuously been posed (see, for example, Indian Council of Medical Research 2000).

However, 1994 was the year of a major global paradigm shift, when infertility was conceptually included into reproductive health programs (Rao 2004, 17). The declaration of the United Nations International Conference on Population and Development, to which India was a signatory, defined reproductive health as "a state of complete physical, mental and social wellbeing, and not merely the absence of disease or infirmity, in all matters relating to the reproductive system and its processes. Reproductive health therefore implies that people are able to have a satisfying and safe sex life and that they have the capability to reproduce and the freedom to decide if, when, and how often to do so" (United Nations Population Fund 2014, 59). This shift accomplished the inclusion of infertility in political agendas and public discourses. Even earlier, India had reoriented its policy focus from "family planning" to "family welfare," which was later followed by the "reproductive and child health program" (National Institute for Research in Reproductive Health, n.d.). It is in this context that public hospitals in India have started to open IVF units since the 2000s, amid a therapeutic terrain that had long been dominated by private providers.

Furthermore, the technologization of infertility management, in particular through IVF, aligned well with predominant forms of solutionism and catapulted reproductive medicine from dusty gynecological offices into the shiny realms of specialized, high-tech biomedicine. Reproductive technologies could now be proudly celebrated as part of India's globalized modernity in a milieu where "biomedicine has become a metonym for modernity in the domain of healing" (Connor 2001, 7). Simultaneously, reproductive technologies have been politically claimed as part of a glorious national past. Politicians in India have declared reproductive medicine to be a century-old practice (Rahman 2014), highlighting the close entanglement of science and medicine with larger nationalistic discourses (Nanda 2016). The appropriation of IVF for political agendas testifies to the affective dimensions of reproductive technologies and their ability to cater to distinct desires and imaginaries.

Moreover, reproductive medicine in India, and IVF in particular, has become highly relevant for its economic productivity. IVF constitutes a paradigmatic example of the "convergence of the life sciences with systems and regimes of capital" (Sunder Rajan 2012, 2): it is not only a thriving medical specialty but also a high-revenue-generating and fast-growing industry (Sama Resource Group for Women and Health 2010; S. Banerjee 2015; Rudrappa 2015). A systematic analysis of health surveys estimated that out of 48.5 million couples worldwide who were unable to have a child, almost one-third (14.4 million) lived in South Asia in 2010 (Mascarenhas et al. 2012). According to a former vice president of the Indian Society for Assisted Reproduction, the use of IVF in India has increased almost six-fold since the turn of the millennium: while in the year 2000 only seven thousand IVF cycles were conducted annually in India, the number has risen to forty thousand cycles per year a decade later (Datta 2010, 38). However, already in the year 2000, the Indian Council of Medical Research estimated that "for a population of one billion approximately 400,000 IVF cycles will need to be performed annually." Further, in contrast to 31 IVF units in the year 2000 (Datta 2010, 38), their number grew to roughly 500 in 2010 and 1,500 in 2019, according to an estimate of the International Federation of Fertility Societies (2019), implying that almost one-fourth of IVF clinics worldwide are currently located in India. The National Registry of Assisted Reproductive Technology (ART) Clinics and Banks in India, which was initiated by the Indian Council of Medical Research, shows that as of April 2021, 542 hospitals have enrolled with the registry, out of which 69 are located in Delhi. Yet it is important to note that statistics are hardly reliable, and estimates range from anywhere between five hundred and thirty thousand assisted reproductive technologies facilities in the country (Bharadwaj 2016, 23).

Ambiguous data allows for promises of spectacular growth. A report published by Ernst and Young (2015, 4), for example, analyzes the IVF market in India not only as "highly fragmented" but also as "highly under-penetrated." On the premise that currently only 1 percent of the twenty-two to thirty-three million infertile couples in India seek infertility interventions, it projects enormous growth rates by observing that "with more infertile couples coming forward for treatment, the IVF market is estimated to grow by about 20 percent to about 260,000 cycles by 2020" (42). The report depicts India as a "new frontier" (Comaroff and Comaroff 2012) in a global medical market, which encourages international investors, national large-scale businesses, and local middlemen to enter the IVF landscape. Furthermore, the country continues to hit the limelight as a destination for transnational medical travel (Kaspar and Reddy 2017), particularly with regard to surrogacy (Pande 2014; Rudrappa 2015; Deomampo 2016; Majumdar 2017; Saravanan 2018), although a newly proposed bill is likely to change this image in the future, since only Indian citizens may be allowed to undergo surrogacy in the country.

Despite this rhetoric of hype, it is important to remember that India's contributions to the making of global reproductive medicine started long before the 2000s and that the country's role has shifted enormously in the process: from a provider of raw material to a producer of knowledge and, subsequently, a thriving medical market that attracts patients from all over the world—a (not quite so linear) trajectory that will be described in the first part of the book. This might be read as a symptom of the transformations in the country's political economy on a broader level: reverberations of British colonialism, a socialist planning economy after Independence in 1947, and economic liberalization programs since the 1980s, are all reflected in the history of reproductive medicine. Although the growth of IVF units in India since the 1990s is certainly due to the increasing medical standardization of the procedure and the realization of gynecologists that "this is not rocket science," as one IVF practitioner put it, it is also based on the country's economic reforms and the subsequent availability of medical and financial infrastructure. Rather than an experimental endeavor, the setup of an IVF center in India nowadays constitutes a relatively solid business opportunity that national investors and global capital are quick to embark on. For instance, Bourn Hall Clinic, the hospital in the United Kingdom that was founded in 1980 by the British researchers who were responsible for the world's first IVF baby, inaugurated its first branch in India in 2011 (*The Hindu* 2011). Taking this economic profitability into account, one could cynically remark that IVF practitioners and investors have successfully appropriated the long-standing feminist claim that reproduction is always also productive (Thompson 2005).

For patients, however, IVF proves to be mostly expensive and sometimes unaffordable. As private insurance providers do not pay for IVF procedures in India, patients in private hospitals have to cover expenses out of pocket. Prices vary according to hospitals, and may range from roughly 80,000 Rs. to almost 200,000 Rs. (between ca. 1,000 and 2,700 USD) for one IVF cycle. While patients in public hospitals receive most procedures for free, they have to provide funding for pharmaceuticals and other disposables (between 20,000 Rs. and 70,000 Rs., or 270 and 940 USD). Only a few low-income workers and government employees can reclaim expenses spent in government hospitals through public insurance programs. Many patients therefore struggled financially to either pay for one IVF cycle or finance their repeated attempts. They used their savings, took up loans from family members and banks, or even sold land and jewelry.

Despite the country's longstanding history of "reproductive governance" (Morgan and Roberts 2012), reproductive technologies are barely subjected to regulation in India. Although infertility management is partly moderated by the *National Guidelines for Accreditation, Supervision and Regulation of ART Clinics in India*, developed by the Indian Council of Medical Research and the Ministry of Health and Family Welfare in 2002 and published in 2005, they are not legally binding. Further, various versions of the Draft Assisted Reproductive Technology (Regulation) Bill (2008, 2010, 2012, 2014, 2015)—documents that aspire to turn some of the regulations posited by the guidelines into law—have been awaiting their debate in Parliament for several years. This decades-long legislative void has resulted in a scarcely monitored sector. However, in February 2020 the Union Cabinet finally approved the bill, and it was introduced in the Lok Sabha (the lower house of the Indian Parliament) on September 14, 2020. It has been referred to a standing committee, whose report was issued on March 19, 2021. In addition to the Assisted Reproductive Technology (Regulation) Bill, 2020, a separate bill for surrogacy has been in preparation since 2016. The 2019 version passed the Lok Sabha and was introduced in the Rajya Sabha (the upper house of the Indian Parliament). The Rajya Sabha referred the bill to a select committee, which "underscored the importance of passing the ART Bill before the Surrogacy Bill" (Banerjee and Kotiswaran 2021, 89) in its report.

Fertile Fields

This book draws on twenty-four months of nonconsecutive fieldwork between 2010 and 2017.[16] To complement the predominantly synchronic accounts about assisted reproductive technologies in India, I conducted oral history research and archival work. Further, in addition to contemporary "negotiated interactive observation" (Wind 2008) and interviews in IVF hospitals in Delhi, I also engaged with policy documents, scientific articles, and reports in magazines and newspapers.

Historical research was carried out in India (Delhi, Kolkata, and Mumbai), the Netherlands, Germany, the United Kingdom, and Switzerland. I conducted oral history research with a variety of interlocutors. In chapter 1, I rely on interviews and informal conversations with former managers and employees of a pharmaceutical company in India and the Netherlands, organizers of a urine collection program in Kolkata, medical representatives, and—with the help of a research assistant—urine donors. In chapter 2, I build on long-term engagements with Dr. Subhas's family members, friends, colleagues, students, and former patients as well as observations at memorial events and conferences. I also spoke to representatives of medical organizations, government officials, politicians, and journalists in Kolkata and Delhi. Chapter 3 is based on interviews with a range of scientists, doctors, and embryologists in the field of reproductive medicine about their clinical careers in India as well as conversations with medical distributors and other entrepreneurs connected to the IVF sector in Delhi, Kolkata, and Mumbai. Further, I draw on records from the National Archives of India, the Nehru Memorial Museum and Library Archives, the National Library of India, and the archives of the National Institute for Research in Reproductive Health. This material was further corroborated by archival work at the Institute for Studies in Industrial Development, the Indian Drug Manufacturers' Association, pharmaceutical companies in the Netherlands and Germany, the Churchill Archives Centre in Cambridge, and the World Health Organization in Geneva. Finally, many interlocutors provided me with gray literature in the form of documents, leaflets, informal publications, and photographs. While the first part of the book is largely based on historical material, the second part relies on long-term ethnographic fieldwork.

In order to investigate the contemporary making of IVF and following Aditya Bharadwaj's (2016, 251) prompt that "IVF clinics in India need to be more systematically examined," I based my fieldwork in two hospitals. In 2009, I sent several emails to IVF practitioners explaining my project and requesting access to their hospitals. A very prominent fertility doctor in Delhi, who herself had a keen interest in research work, invited me for an initial meeting and later allowed me to conduct long-term research within the premises of her private hospital. She had opened one of the first IVF centers in the city in the 1990s, and at the time of my fieldwork there (2010 and 2012), she both owned and administered this hospital, which I call PremiumIVF. With over eleven million inhabitants (and over sixteen million in the National Capital Region), Delhi is one of the most populous cities in India. Providing an array of tertiary care services, the city attracts patients from different states across India. Apart from a few exceptions, Delhi's IVF hospitals cater mainly to an Indian (and sometimes nonresident Indian) patient population (for the necessity to examine IVF as a procedure used by Indian patients, see Singh 2017). This stands in contrast to centers in West India (e.g., Gujarat and Mumbai) that used to specifically target international patients for surrogacy services (e.g., Vora 2013; Pande 2014; Deomampo 2016; Saravanan 2018). In addition to a diverse landscape of private clinics, Delhi also housed two out of the formerly three public IVF hospitals in the country as well as a unit run by the Indian Army. Since I also had the opportunity to observe daily clinical life in one of Delhi's government hospitals, this constitutes the first ethnography in India of what Kate Hampshire and Bob Simpson (2015) have called "assisted reproductive technologies in the third phase," a phase during which these technologies have become available and are accessible to wider segments of the population. After I had met the responsible clinicians at conferences in 2012, I obtained their permission to spend time in the IVF unit of a public hospital, which I call CommonCare. "Deep hanging out" (Rosaldo 1989) in different clinical contexts enabled me to examine IVF practice not only as it is represented in medical textbooks, official documents, during conferences, or in formal interviews, but also as it presented itself in "action" (Latour 1987).

During my stay, both IVF centers fully concentrated on fertility-related interventions and had a rather high patient load for Delhi (around forty IVF cycles per month). In addition to IVF, they conducted other diagnostic and therapeutic procedures, such as laparoscopy, hysteroscopy, ovulation induction, intrauterine insemination (IUI), intracytoplasmic sperm injection (ICSI), surrogacy, and so on.[17] At both centers, I observed everyday realities of clinical life in various spaces: the consultation room, the ultrasound room, the operation theater, the embryology laboratory, and patients' recovery rooms. I witnessed several hundred medical procedures, acquired basic medical knowledge, and learned the technical language of the field.[18] While I had unrestricted access and was provided with a doctor's dress (clinical hierarchies are discernable in sartorial arrangements), I remained a bystander during medical procedures. In consultations, which happened in closed rooms in PremiumIVF and in more open arrangements in CommonCare, I sat in a chair at the short side of the consultation table where doctors and patients were seated and faced each other, but I usually remained silent. My active participation in the hospital was reserved for more informal situations: lunch breaks, tea sessions, or chats during the slower parts of the day.

As Marcia Inhorn (2004, 2096) states, it is indeed quite challenging "when those who are not physicians attempt to penetrate the hospital clinic in order to apply an 'ethnographic gaze on the medical gaze' (in part to examine structures of power)." This was aggravated by the fact that I was "studying up" (Nader 1972) in terms of class and professional career, at least in relation to physicians.[19] Many clinicians were perplexed at first that I, as a social anthropologist, was also interested in their work instead of only the social characteristics and cultural understandings of their patients. In order to turn medical practice into an object of inquiry, it was therefore necessary to conduct long-term fieldwork and try to become part of clinical life.

While I spent many hours a day with doctors observing clinical routines, I also spent much time at patients' bedsides, asking them about their experiences in nonmedical terms. I conducted semistructured, open-ended interviews in English or Hindi with ninety patients and sometimes their attendants (usually husbands, mothers, or mothers-in-law) in both IVF centers. I was introduced to patients as a researcher, an observer, or a student from abroad.[20] With some people, I conducted repeat interviews over a period of several years outside the hospital, either in their homes or in places of their choice. Consent was granted orally, and interviews were recorded on tape or in writing.[21] Since I promised anonymity to participants, I either use pseudonyms or refer to them generically as "patients."[22]

Most of the patients I spoke to were female, although their husbands or partners sometimes took part in conversations (for a different perspective, see Inhorn 2012). They were from various parts of India and of different socioeconomic standing. The majority of my interlocutors was Hindu, but I also encountered Muslim and Christian IVF users. While I could easily negotiate access as a woman, as a foreign, white researcher I was clearly a stranger for most interlocutors. This strangeness, however, was usually met with sympathy and curiosity. People were interested in the ways in which IVF is conducted in Germany and enthusiastically engaged in comparative endeavors. A few patients also hoped to receive advice about hospitals and contacts to doctors—expectations that I tried to fulfill to the best of my abilities. Finally, my strangeness provided a sense of anonymity. Some interlocutors told me that they found it quite helpful to tell their stories to a person outside their social circles who is not a doctor but familiar with IVF and who has time to listen (Inhorn 2004; Whittaker 2015).

Even though I started with a "hospital ethnography" (van der Geest and Finkler 2004) and was indeed grounded in two IVF clinics, it was nevertheless necessary to account for the fact that hospitals are "simultaneously bounded and permeable" spaces (Street and Coleman 2012, 4). It was therefore crucial for me to meet clinicians as well as patients not only in their professional roles or in their personae as medical subjects. I was on cordial terms with several junior doctors and interacted with them in their free time. I saw how some of them started their own clinics and how they have now become established members of the IVF community in Delhi. I also became friends with some patients, who I met with regularly over several years. Following their trajectory, long after they had left the hospital, gave me invaluable insights into their dealings with an intimate and often agonizing process and allowed me to contextualize infertility and IVF as part of everyday lives.

Additionally, I followed various trails to other fertile fields (for "multi-sited ethnography," see Marcus 1995): from the various institutions offering IVF in Delhi to an embryology training course in Mumbai, from conferences and educational sessions to the offices of policy makers and politicians, from counseling rooms to patients' homes, from the homes of gamete donors to donor agencies. Although they have informed my view on reproductive medicine in India, I decided to largely exclude the experiences of gamete donors, surrogates, and agencies, as they have already received extensive public attention and scholarly treatment, to which I refer interested readers (Vora 2013; Pande 2014; Reddy and Patel 2015; Rudrappa 2015; Tanderup et al. 2015; Deomampo 2016; Majumdar 2017; Bärnreuther 2018, 2020; B. Parry 2018; Saravanan 2018). Instead, the principal contribution of the present book lies in providing an analysis of IVF as a mundane medical intervention, as it has been in the making in India.

The Chapters to Come

This book examines the making of global reproductive medicine in postcolonial India with a focus on IVF. In the first part (chapters 1 to 3), I trace the genealogy of India's position within the field of reproductive medicine from the 1960s up to the present day. Following the transnational flows of bodily material, knowledge claims, medical supplies, and financial investments, I highlight India's substantial but shifting role in shaping global reproductive medicine: from a provider of raw material to a producer of knowledge to a thriving medical market. This part of the book provides insight into the political-economic relations on which global reproductive medicine has relied and through which the IVF sector in India has begun to thrive.

In chapter 1, I follow the commodity chain of a pharmaceutical substance used in infertility management: hCG, a hormone derived from pregnant women's urine. Between the 1960s and 1990s, an extensive urine collection scheme was established among the urban poor in Kolkata to supply the European pharmaceutical industry with biological raw material for the production of hCG. Promises of productivity in terms of fertility and development enabled extractive mechanisms at a time when India's political economy was characterized by protectionism and policies of self-sufficiency. The alchemy of hCG from a seemingly impotent waste product in India to a productive pharmaceutical commodity in Europe relied on a racialized, classed, and gendered set of relations that has long sustained global reproductive medicine. While this story fits the familiar narrative of extraction of raw material from the global South to the global North, the next chapter complicates this view.

In chapter 2, I continue to investigate transnational entanglements through a connecting figure: Dr. Subhas Mukherjee, a reproductive biologist who worked as a consultant for the urine collection program. In 1978, the same year as the first IVF baby was born in the United Kingdom, he claimed that he too had created a "test-tube baby" in Kolkata. The claim was later dismissed, as it constituted what I call an "innovation out of place": the experiments were conducted outside the laboratory, institutional structures, scientific conventions, and established centers of innovation. Contrary to the biological material described in chapter 1, this knowledge claim could not flow unhindered but faced severe barriers in its reach. However, starting from the late 1990s, Dr. Subhas's achievements have become recognized, at least among medical circles in India. And it is this surprising shift that the chapter unravels: How did Dr. Subhas's proposition turn into a fact two decades later although medical evidence had not changed? I argue that this transformation was rendered possible by shifts in the perception of legitimate spaces of innovation. For reasons that are the subject of the next chapter, India could now be imagined as a place that innovations emerge from rather than diffuse to.

In chapter 3, I examine the formation of a transnational fertility market and an uneven field of medical providers in contemporary Delhi. Drawing on in-depth interviews with crucial stakeholders, such as clinical pioneers who practiced in the private and public sectors, I describe the rise of IVF as a thriving medical specialty and high-revenue-generating industry. In addition to postcolonial health care policy, it was the economic reforms in India that contributed to the transformation of IVF between the 1980s and 2000s: from a public research project to a largely privatized practice; from a "hobby" undertaken by inventive doctors to a commercialized object of consumption; from an improvised, experimental procedure to a routinized, standardized intervention. However, these shifts do not constitute linear developments: public hospitals, for instance, have offered IVF since 2008. The chapter proposes that this is but one example of how the public and private, the experimental and standardized, the improvised and materially stable blend into each other. The interplay and tension between these spheres have culminated in a stratified field, which results in diverse treatment options and unequal access to services.

In the second part of the book (chapters 4 to 6), I examine the contemporary making of IVF in hospitals and laboratories in Delhi. Focusing on everyday realities of clinical life, I zoom in on the objects of clinical practice, such as bodies, gametes, and embryos. I argue that making IVF work means working on and with reproductive substances in conjunction with technologies, pharmaceuticals, protocols, and guidelines. For example, clinicians attempt to turn bodies designated as infertile into productive entities, make acceptable gametes that are understood to be improper, and manipulate embryos considered to be unpredictable. Yet, despite these efforts, experiences of failure, anxiety, and uncertainty remain dominant in IVF hospitals.

In chapter 4, I depict how patients navigate the stratified clinical landscape in Delhi in their quest to establish substantial relations and create their "own" offspring. Patients maneuver a terrain of continuous promises and frequent failures that constantly involves decision-making, attempts to deal with uncertainties, and adjustments to setbacks. Over the course of the chapter, five women recount their shifting relations to infertility management in general and IVF in particular. In addition to analyzing patients'—often cyclical—relationship to IVF, the chapter also serves as an introduction to the clinical part of the IVF process, in which further dimensions of temporality come into play. I describe how IVF cycles unfold over time and how time is calibrated when bodily rhythms are regulated on the one hand and medical interventions ordered around bodily temporalities on the other.

Although IVF may be able to create desired connections, it also carries the danger of generating unwanted ties, as I discuss in chapter 5. Since reproductive substances are imbued with the ability to establish substantial relations, their seemingly uncontrolled movement in IVF laboratories elicits fears and suspicions about mismatches and mix-ups among patients. Mixing gametes, a process that is essential for reproduction, goes hand in hand with anxieties of adulteration, for example when biological substances move to realms outside kinship, caste, or religious groups. Exploring the stratified circulations of gametes in different hospitals, I show how patients and medical professionals navigate IVF as a procedure that constantly threatens social norms. Finally, I analyze how rumors about mix-ups overlap with wider discourses of sociomoral degeneration and interpret them as critical commentaries on present social transformations in urban, capitalist India.

After highlighting the ability of substances to establish relations—whether desired or not, I argue in chapter 6 that substances themselves are constituted relationally. Turning to the laboratory, I discuss how embryologists manage prevailing experiences of unpredictability by trying to control embryos on the one hand and carefully tending to their needs on the other. The fact that embryos remain indeterminate raises not only epistemological questions but also ethical ones. I describe how embryologists' "ethical judgment" (Lambek 1997) of embryos either as living beings or as relational entities permeates daily laboratory practice. The chapter demonstrates that although biologicals are certainly able to generate and define relations, they, in turn, are "matter related" (Abrahamsson et al. 2015), made through and situated within very specific sociopolitical, technological, legislative, and ethical relations.

FROM URINE TO AMPOULE

The Commodity Chain of a Hormone

"Are you going to be a mother?" (*Āpni ki mā hate calechen?*) This question was inscribed on a billboard captured in a slightly blurred photograph that Mr. Velden was showing me in his living room in a small town in the Netherlands. It was part of a photo album depicting his visits to India. As a former representative of a biochemical company, Mr. Velden had overseen a urine collection program in Kolkata. The billboard in the photograph had been erected close to the entrance of the company grounds in the outskirts of the city. Its inscription invited pregnant women to help their infertile contemporaries by donating urine, which contains human chorionic gonadotropin (hCG). The semiprocessed urine would then be transported by air to Oss, an industrial town in the Netherlands, where Mr. Velden's company purified it to manufacture a pharmaceutical that was sold internationally for infertility management. Tracing hCG's "commodity chain" (Hopkins and Wallerstein 1986) between the 1960s and 1990s allows me to explore the alchemy of this hormone from a seemingly impotent waste product in Kolkata to a productive pharmaceutical commodity in the Netherlands.[1] Or as Bruno Lunenfeld, a scientist who was instrumental in this field (see below), put it: hCG's transformation from "urine into gold" (quoted in Livneh 2002). This alchemy was facilitated by promises of productivity that made the fertility of the urban poor in the global South available and valuable for reproductive medicine in the global North.

In this chapter, I explore in detail the conditions of possibility that enabled the making of hCG, not only as a pharmaceutical but also as an important

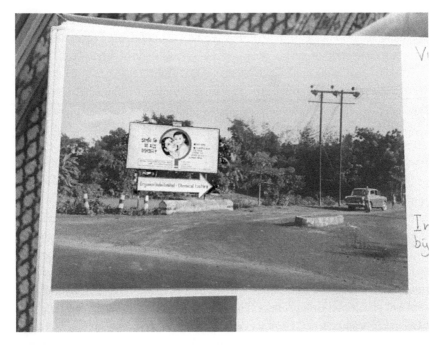

FIGURE 2. Photo of a billboard in Mr. Velden's photo album. Photo by the author.

techno-scientific infrastructure for global reproductive medicine. Until the 1990s, IVF hospitals all over the world would prescribe "urinary hCG" for medical procedures. Today, many hospitals in low-income countries still use urinary hCG instead of newer and costlier recombinant pharmaceuticals. However, the substantial relations between pregnant and infertile women in different parts of the world are neither detectable in the final product nor communicated in the hospital. Making the relations congealed in this pharmaceutical legible not only highlights minute processes of valuation that go beyond biological extraction and chemical metamorphosis but also emphasizes the vital role of India for the global reproductive industry.

Hormonal Alchemy

hCG is a hormone or, to be more exact, one of three gonadotropins, which control gamete and sex hormone production.[2] hCG specifically is secreted by the placenta during pregnancy. hCG is also an essential pharmaceutical for infertility management. When administered medically, it promotes follicular maturation and induces ovulation in female patients. Furthermore, hCG can be employed to advance fertility in male and animal bodies. In its off-label uses, hCG has been applied quite creatively, for example for weight loss. Until the 1980s, the production of hCG as a pharmaceutical required the biochemical extraction of the active ingredient from pregnant women's urine.[3] It therefore relied heavily on human raw material that was sourced in various parts of the world. Kolkata was one of these places.

The fact that India specifically, or the global South more generally, has long served as a source for bodily extraction is well-known (Cohen 2005). Noteworthy, however, are the alchemical moments built into the commodity chain of hCG. In this chapter, I analyze hCG's transformation from somatic source as urine to packaged product as ampoules. Apart from biochemical mutations—the changes in the form of the substance itself—the transformation of hCG was achieved through processes of valuation. Encompassing valorization as well as evaluation (Vatin 2013), processes of valuation, I argue, relied on specific relational constellations. Among them were alliances between academy and industry in Europe; cooperation between India and the Netherlands; and, most important, connections between pregnant and infertile women. Depicting these constellations allows me to make visible the racialized, classed, and gendered set of relations that underlay the commodity chain of hCG but was no longer detectable in the final pharmaceutical product. Thus, similar to other capitalist commodities, hCG as a pharmaceutical product came "into value by using—and obviating—non-capitalist social relations" (Tsing 2013, 21; see also Sunder Rajan 2006, 41). Further, I argue that the commodity chain of hCG was not only "animated by multiple, layered and complex interactions between material objects and structural relations of production" but also by "abstractions" (Sunder Rajan 2006, 20) or conjurations of promissory futures (Sunder Rajan, 119). In the case of hCG, visions of a productive future in the form of somatic fertility and economic development helped to enroll the urban poor, medical doctors in Kolkata, and the Indian state into the urine collection program. Most important, they enabled extractive mechanisms at a time when India's political economy was characterized by protectionism and policies of self-sufficiency. In this sense, hCG "yoked" (Haraway 2012, 307) not only pregnant and infertile bodies but also postcolonial landscapes in the global South and thriving bioeconomies in the global North. Promises of somatic and economic fertility proved to be powerful and productive, although most were never realized.

Fertile Relations

I analyze the multilayered relational constellations on which the commodity chain of hCG was based in three steps: hCG's industrial production was made possible through the entanglement of academy and industry during the first half of the twentieth century, which consolidated European pharmaceutical companies as we know them today. The internationalization of one of these companies in the 1960s contributed to the establishment of relations between India and the Netherlands through the externalization of supply chains. It is in this context that Kolkata became a site where pregnant women donated urine for infertile contemporaries all over the world.

Between Academy and Industry

During the first half of the twentieth century, researchers tried to turn hCG and other gonadotropins into clinically applicable products. In order to do so, scientists had to cooperate with pharmaceutical companies, as only they were able to initiate large-scale collection programs for raw material, industrialize the extraction procedure, manufacture products, and conduct clinical trials (Bettendorf 1995, 360). However, there used to be practical concerns regarding the collaboration between academy and industry.[4] Bruno Lunenfeld, who was a central figure in gonadotropin research and part of the so-called G-Club—a club that had been founded in the name of gonadotropins in 1953—remembered his meeting with the board of directors of Serono in 1958.[5] He tried to convince Serono, an Italian pharmaceutical company at that time, to enter the field of hMG (human menopausal gonadotropin) production, a hormonal preparation extracted from the urine of postmenopausal women.[6]

> So I presented our data to the board of directors of Serono, they applauded me, but claimed they were not a "pissoire," and that seemed the end of my dreams. However, as we left, a member of the board approached me, and Dr Donini [Pietro Donini, a senior scientist at Serono at that time] introduced him as Prince Pacelli. He invited me to stay in Rome and we met every day for a week, when he called the board back and gave them a similar lecture to mine, but ending with: "My uncle, the Pope, has made arrangements for the collection of urine in the old age homes of nuns and will donate this urine." It turned out that the bank Banco di Santo Spirito of the Vatican owned Serono shares, which is why Prince Pacelli was on the Serono board. (Lunenfeld 2009, 37; see also Lunenfeld 2013, 14)

In the end, Prince Giulio Pacelli, an Italian aristocrat, initiated Serono's industrial production of hMG with the help of Pope Pius XII and about three hundred Italian nuns—a quite surprising, if not to say unholy, alliance in the field of reproductive medicine.[7]

The collaboration between academy and industry also unfolded in terms of hCG production in one of the other prominent "hormone companies" in Europe: Organon. Organon was founded in the Netherlands in 1923 through another unlikely alliance: between Saal van Zwanenberg, the owner of a slaughterhouse; Ernst Laqueur, a professor of pharmacology at the University of Amsterdam; and Jacques van Oss, a chemist and consultant for Van Zwanenberg. While Van Zwanenberg was looking for a profitable way to get rid of his slaughterhouse's waste products, Laqueur required glands for research on gonadal hormones (Oudshoorn 1994, 69). The collaboration between slaughterhouse and laboratory effectively joined the provision of raw material and scientific expertise, although it remained largely invisible to consumers who "would not be able to identify the link between Zwan's smoked sausage and Organon's contraceptive pill" (Verhoog 1998, 14). The cooperation continued to work profitably for both parties even after the source for many hormones shifted to urine as raw material (Oudshoorn 1994, 71).

After Organon had started its urine collection program for hCG production in the Netherlands in 1931, men in black suits, called *pismannekes* ("small piss men" in Dutch), used to retrieve the substance from pregnant women's homes, stopping their bicycles or horse carriages at houses with a newspaper placed on the windowsill. The women were mobilized by bakers, midwives, or nurses and later by specifically recruited ambassadors (Moeders voor Moeders, n.d.a). Since 1966, the program has been running under a new name: Moeders voor Moeders (Mothers for Mothers in Dutch; Tausk 1984, 31).[8] Volunteers have not been paid much for their contributions, but an early information brochure of Moeders voor Moeders states that "each participant receives a compensation and an appropriate gift for the effort made" (Moeders voor Moeders, n.d.b, my translation).[9]

Organon's history is just one account of how scientific research and industrial production were conjoined in pharmaceutical companies in Europe during the first half of the twentieth century. Jean-Paul Gaudillière (2005, 641) calls this move an "internalization of biology": "During the years 1930–1950, the major pharmaceutical companies took decisive steps in the direction of developing their own, in-house biological research infrastructure." When the demand for gonadotropins increased considerably, particularly after their clinical application in the 1960s and their regular use in reproductive medicine since the 1980s (Practice Committee of the American Society for Reproductive Medicine 2008, S13), this internalization of biology was complemented by the externalization of supply chains, a strategy that was closely linked to Organon's increasing global operations: after a McKinsey report in 1963 advised "internationalization," Organon opened subsidiaries all over the world to sell its products (Verhoog 1998, 9, 68). Further, it also extended its search for raw material abroad. It was this quest for new markets and resources that brought the company to Kolkata.

Between Europe and India

A booklet depicting a brief history of Organon India states that the company had "reached the Indian shores in 1961."[10] After a brief alliance with Martin & Harris, a British pharmaceutical company, Organon (India) Limited was formed and registered on August 30, 1967.[11] The fact that Organon only distributed imported pharmaceuticals at first reflected the state of India's pharmaceutical sector in the 1960s and early 1970s, where MNCs (multinational companies) controlled large shares of the market but operated mainly through import. "The Indian pharmaceutical market remained import-dependent through the 1960s until the government-initiated policies stressing self-reliance through local production" (Mazumdar 2013, 19). These policies included the elimination of product patents through the Patents Act 1970, changes to the Foreign Exchange Regulation Act 1973, and the introduction of the New Drug Policy in 1978 (Chaudhuri 2005, 37). Apart from restrictions on imports of ready-made products, the Indian government required MNCs to locally produce bulk drugs (i.e., active pharmaceutical ingredients) in order to promote industrial development and reduce import dependency (Chaudhuri 2005). According to former employees, these regulations forced Organon to open manufacturing facilities in India.[12] In the early 1970s, Organon thus inaugurated two production sites in Kolkata: one for pharmaceutical items and another for bulk drugs. In 1974, the company applied for an industrial license with the Indian government to manufacture steroids and export hCG.

Between the Fertile and the Infertile

Organon India was asked to produce hCG in the early 1970s, at a time when demand increased worldwide. According to my interlocutors in the Netherlands, it was feared that the supply of pregnant women's urine from the Netherlands would cease to be sufficient.[13] In its industrial license application to the Government of India in 1974, Organon India therefore specified its need for urine as raw material. Referring to the large population and high birth rates in India, it was rather confident about its ability to collect the needed amount. "The raw material required for the purpose is at the moment a total waste in the country. Further availability of the raw material is plenty, for which large scale manufacturing of this product and its different preparations are possible without any difficulty" (National Archives of India 1977). Ironically, while the size and growth rate of India's population had usually been conceptualized as hindering economic development during those decades, it was precisely these factors that were now turned into a precious resource to be harvested by a multinational company.

But urine collection did not run as smoothly as imagined. Dr. Chatterjee, a former manager of Organon India, who was entrusted with a pilot project to examine the feasibility of hCG production, recounted how he was overwhelmed with this unusual task: "They wanted me to do something about hCG. hCG comes from first trimester pregnant urine. . . . I am a Brahmin, working with urine was not my job. I am a synthetic drug man. . . . That was my line. Steroids, that was my line. My line was not handling urine." While he was familiar with the production of synthetic hormones, he felt repulsed and unequipped to extract hormones from raw material, and even more so from urine, a smelly and polluting substance.[14] Dr. Chatterjee's concerns were mainly tied to his status as a high-caste and educated employee.[15] However, his friend Dr. Subhas Mukherjee, a clinician and researcher (see chapter 2; Bärnreuther 2016), who also acted as a consultant to Organon India, encouraged him to engage with the project and helped him organize the collection.

In the beginning, Dr. Chatterjee and Dr. Subhas tried to enroll residents of high-income areas: "The first suggestion was to request friends from Ballygunge [an upper-middle-class neighborhood] to donate, because they are the ones who get to know that they are pregnant early [at a time when pregnancy tests were rare]," Dr. Chatterjee explained. "But in the end, they would not donate, because people would ask why does this car come every day and collect bottles? So, this failed." After middle-class propriety and social surveillance had thwarted their plans, both agreed that Dr. Chatterjee, who was a former general secretary of Jadavpur University's student union and considered a "people's man," should go to North Kolkata, "to poor people's villages" and ask for assistance there. And indeed, they slowly began to succeed in convincing women in these areas to participate in the collection program.

In addition to logistical challenges to collecting urine, a racialized and classed understanding of biology created apprehensions about the potency of urine from the urban poor in Kolkata. As Dr. Chatterjee detailed, "We did not know whether we will get hCG. Some funny idea was there whether poor Indian women would have hCG. . . . Initially we were afraid whether we will get it at all." Yet in the end, both concerns proved to be unfounded: the company managed to collect urine in large quantities and was able to extract hCG from it. Dr. Chatterjee gave an impression of how the collection program started off under his direction: "With permission from the company we organized monthly meetings in every center and the mothers were given small presents. . . . We collected 100 to 200 liters per day. Later maybe more, but I only stayed for five and a half years." And indeed, in 1980 the collection had reached around eight hundred liters per day (*Statesman* 1980). It may have gone up to three thousand or four thousand liters per day, according to an estimate by

Mr. Banerjee, the acquisition manager of hCG, who was responsible for the program after Dr. Chatterjee had left the company. Mr. Banerjee expanded the collection area by incorporating wider regions in the district. He described donors as mostly labor class, many of them migrants, and more than half of them Muslims. According to Mr. Banerjee the fact that families tended to be large (hence the opportunity to recruit women during several pregnancies) turned these areas into "fertile grounds for collection."

After the program had been popularized, women who had missed their menstrual period knew that they would have to call a so-called ladyworker responsible for their neighborhood to get tested. In case of a positive outcome, women would be notified about their pregnancy. The collection regime would start immediately, lasting until week sixteen of the pregnancy. Each morning, collection boys would bring a plastic bottle containing a preservative while picking up the filled bottle they had left the day before.[16] The boys would transport the urine by bicycle to one of the collection centers, from where a company cart would bring the bottles to the factory. Once the collection was over, urine donors received a small present (*upahār*).

The gift handed over after the collection was described by Dr. Chatterjee as "something useful" and "not very costly because the benefit ratio has to be kept." Initially this used to be Horlick powder, a powdered milk drink produced by another MNC, which was advertised to a middle-class audience in India at that time with the slogan "the great nourisher." Providing Horlick powder seems quite fitting: future mothers, who care for their infertile sisters by giving a substance, receive another substance to care for their own children. It can be read as a symbol for the nourishing relationship that the slogan "mothers for mothers" promises. Yet, at second glance, it completely neglects the inequalities involved in this exchange. As former employees reported, many donors sold their Horlick powder to buy rice instead, which they evidently deemed more nourishing for their families. After complaints from regular Horlick retailers that the powder was being sold under market value, Organon India changed its presents to household appliances, such as buckets, steel plates, or jugs.

Promises of Productivity

Corporeal Generosity through the Promise of Somatic Fertility

But how did Organon India convince pregnant women to donate urine? Apart from handing out small presents, no payments were provided to participants because the company was afraid that "men would also contribute," as had apparently happened in other countries before.[17] Instead, Organon India relied on women's corporeal generosity,[18] as Dr. Chatterjee explained: "We never talked about money. It was only an appeal. You know, Indian women are very kind in heart. . . . No money was provided. It was not money exchange; it was only people helping." But women may not only have been willing to donate out of altruism—particularly since urine collection raised concerns, as an official interviewed by the *Statesman*, a leading English-language newspaper, explained at that time: "Referring to the constraint in implementing the project, the official says many families do not like to be associated with the project. There are elderly people in some families who harbour the erroneous belief that donation of urine may harm the child" (*Statesman* 1980). Mrs. Roy, a former ladyworker, also detailed in a conversation with me how some women or their families would decline to participate in the program because they considered the procedure harmful (*kṣatikārak*) or shameful (*lajjār*). However, not everyone might have felt comfortable to refuse when asked by a doctor or ladyworker, considering the hierarchical relations that characterize the health care sector in India. Further, giving urine had the advantage that women could ascertain whether they were pregnant or not at an early stage. For instance, Mrs. Roy described how some older women would take advantage of the free test to get to know whether their periods had stopped because of menopause or another pregnancy.

For Mrs. Lakshman, who used to be a urine donor and today works in a factory producing packaging material, several motivations converged: when she and her husband moved into a new flat not far from her husband's small blacksmith shop in the 1980s, her landlord introduced her to the program during her first pregnancy. Even though she never ended up receiving a present, she donated her urine again a few years later. Being a good-hearted (*bhālo man*) person—as she described herself and Bengalis in general—she agreed to donate a substance that is usually "thrown away" to help others. Mrs. Lakshman thus reiterated the company's discourse of generous women and worthless substances. In her case, corporeal generosity mainly rested upon the promise of fertility—a gift that she as a future mother could pass on to infertile contemporaries via the company.

In order to emphasize the directionality of the gift toward infertile women, Organon India transferred the slogan "mothers for mothers" into Bengali (*māyer jany mā*) and explained: "if you give urine for a lady who is infertile, she may have a child." According to my interlocutors, this was further corroborated by audiovisual material shown to possible donors that vividly represented the fertile trajectory of their urine: from the jar in their home, to the factory, and finally the doctor's office where an infertile woman is prescribed an ampoule of Pregnyl, the end product. Ladyworkers also made this connection explicit when they motivated women to donate. Mrs. Roy recounted how she would tell potential donors that urine can be transformed from something useless (*akājer*) in the toilet to something beneficial (*phāydā*) in the company's bottle. Similar to blood donation recruiters, ladyworkers argued "not [only] that one is giving one's waste but that not giving is wasteful" (Copeman and Banerjee 2019, 140). The promise of somatic fertility proved to be persuasive. Tapping into cultural valuations of motherhood and geared toward mutuality and solidarity, it resembled the leitmotif that adorns the Dutch Mothers for Mothers website today: "you can share happiness" (*geluk kun je delen* in the Dutch original). The power of the slogan "mothers for mothers" became obvious when Dutch donors threatened to boycott the collection program in the Netherlands after it was made public that hCG can also be used for other purposes, such as weight loss or livestock breeding (Trommelen 2013). Hence, it was the (imagined) bond between pregnant and infertile women that remained essential to donors and, thus, to maintaining supplies.

While this bond proved to be useful during the collection period, it had to be cut later in order to avoid potential economic demands. Framing transactions as generous donations, providing return gifts, and labeling urine as an unproductive substance were important steps in the valorization process of hCG. Discourses of donation obscured the bodily work of donors (Cooper and Waldby 2014) and allowed Organon to evade possible expectations for compensation. The present provided by the company as a return gift further prevented future claims by completing the transaction. Finally, designating bodily substances as waste "free[d] them up for innovative and profitable forms of circulation and transformation" (Waldby and Mitchell 2006, 28). Particularly the rhetoric of *raw* material obfuscated that urine was fertile not only in somatic but also in economic terms. It would eventually turn into corporate wealth, a fact that was not publicized among donors in India. This implied that hCG in its pharmaceutical form reached consumers as an abstract product without any traces of the urine donors who were instrumental for its production (for commodity fetishism, see Marx [1867] 1990).

Public Generosity through the Promise of Economic Development

In addition to donors, various other actors were mobilized through promises revolving around the semantic field of productivity. Organon India employees, for example, harbored the hope that the company would become a "great nourisher" for the pharmaceutical sector specifically and the state of West

Bengal more generally. Envisioning a landscape that had suffered from centuries of colonial rule to become economically fertile again, Organon employees in India were highly invested in the collection program. As in other parts of the world, science generated the "fantasy of regenerating economies devastated by economic restructuring" (Anagnost 2006, 525). A former managing director of Organon India, Mr. Dasgupta, explained to me that he and his colleagues were delighted to set up "something great in West Bengal, where nothing was growing." To turn the region into a fertile field for investment, so to speak. And they even mobilized public resources to do so. According to a report in the *Statesman* (1980), "[t]he West Bengal Government has directed hospitals and health centers in Calcutta and parts of the adjoining districts to help make the private sector project a success." The company enrolled a wide support network of politicians, state officials, and doctors who promoted urine donation by appearing on stage during recruitment events, making sure the program ran smoothly, and calling attention to pregnant women.

Beyond economic reasoning, there was an affective dimension at play, as the manufacture of pharmaceuticals was understood to be a patriotic project in line with broader postcolonial policies pursuing self-sufficiency and self-reliance. Dr. Chatterjee, for instance, told me that Dr. Subhas Mukherjee persuaded him to join the project with the words "[T]his is something India has not done yet. We have to do it. It is your golden opportunity to do it for the country." They were proud of India's joining the ranks of countries that produced hCG. This ethos was apparent in many conversations with former employees in India. They depicted themselves and the company as pioneers who kept the nation's best interest at heart by working for scientific progress and economic development, particularly after the company's "Indianization" (see endnote 12).

The participating gynecologists viewed the company's arrival as an opportunity to improve infertility care and boost their clinical practice. They helped Organon India because they were hoping that the pharmaceutical material they required for clinical procedures and research, especially in the realm of infertility, would become more easily available in India. This was particularly urgent; because of laborious and costly import procedures, most doctors had to procure gonadotropins during trips abroad and smuggle them into the country (see chapter 3; Neveling 2014).

For the state, Organon's presence promised availability of drugs, foreign exchange earnings, and new employment opportunities. In its application for an industrial license in 1974, which included the manufacture of eleven steroids and their formulations as well as hCG and its different preparations, Organon argued that these were "essential drugs where the indigenous manufacturing is not enough to cater to the needs of the market" (National Archives of India

1977). The production of drugs would not only increase their local availability but also promote foreign exchange. The application projected a total foreign exchange earning of almost 32,000,000 Rs. over the course of five years for all products, roughly two-thirds of which were expected to derive from import substitution and one-third from export earnings. Finally, the company promised the "direct employment of over 300 people." Organon concluded its application with the observation that "the dual national objectives of growth of employment and conservation/generation of scarce Foreign Exchange are being met by the Company" (ibid.)—important goals of the Indian government at that time.

And not to forget, Organon also produced gynecological products that were in line with state-sponsored population control programs, such as the contraceptive pill. Both fields, population control and infertility management, have been closely aligned historically. In their license application, for example, Organon specified two clinical uses of hCG: as infertility management in women and men on the one hand and as an "immunological test for early and reliable diagnosis of pregnancy" (ibid.) on the other hand. And indeed, Dr. Subhas Mukherjee was not only interested in hCG for infertility management. He apparently hoped that it would result in the dissemination of home pregnancy tests, for which the company in the Netherlands had obtained the first patent in 1969. In his opinion, this would contribute to population control and ultimately lead to economic development in India.[19] As Dr. Chatterjee recounted,

> Subhas was a nationalist; he was a scientist. He wanted that pregnancy tests should be available from the government to every person. He wanted the family planning program to succeed. He said that population is one of our main problems. Ultimately, population control, you can only do it when you know that you are pregnant. And for knowing it you need pregnancy test kits. And hCG is needed for making pregnancy tests. That's why he wanted it to happen in India. That's why he wanted that hCG is made, so that they can make the kits. He could think far ahead of other people. Commercially, it was a commercial idea. But ideologically it was for reducing pregnancy in India.[20]

It is not surprising then that one of the conditions the Government of India posed in response to Organon's license application was the local production of pregnancy test kits after the first two years. In sum, visions of a productive future in the form of either somatic fertility or economic development helped to enroll the urban poor, medical doctors in Kolkata, and even the Indian state into a scheme organized by an MNC at a time when India's political economy was characterized by protectionism and policies of self-sufficiency.

Unfulfilled Hopes

Commercial Flows

The actual commercial flows, however, contradicted many of the hopes associated with the urine collection program in India. Or, to put it in Dr. Chatterjee's words, commercial goals overruled ideological ones. In 1974, Organon India began to extract hCG from urine of pregnant women, and starting from 1975, crude hCG was exported to the Netherlands.[21] This implies that formulation production did not take place in India and that the exported substance was not fully purified. The final purification and manufacture of the branded pharmaceutical happened in the Netherlands. Moreover, ampoules of the finished product, Pregnyl, were introduced in India only ten years later and were still "too expensive for people here," as Mrs. Roy, the former ladyworker, observed. Further, in contrast to the statement in the license application, pregnancy tests were not produced in Kolkata, as this required hCG of the highest quality. Organon began manufacturing and marketing its pregnancy test, Pregcolor, in India only in 1986. Hence, the hopes harbored by parties who tried to improve infertility management and population control remained largely unfulfilled.

My interlocutors speculated that one reason why the final purification of hCG did not happen in India was that Organon was not prepared to equip the factory in Kolkata with the necessary technologies and know-how. Mr. Banerjee explained that "if they would purify it here . . . Organon would not have full control, they would not be the sole authority. With the crude method, everything is controlled from Holland." In this way, Organon could remain the *"jamidār"* (landlord). Mr. Velden, in contrast, emphasized the requirement of labor power. While the collection in India relied on a large workforce, the last step of purification in the Netherlands could easily be accomplished by a handful of people. In any case, Organon could rely on material resources and cheap labor from India while remaining in control of the production process.

When some of my interlocutors confronted the company with the question of why hCG was not fully purified in India, they received the following answer: "impurity."[22] One IVF doctor, who used to support Organon's collection program in India, remembered that company representatives blamed the Indian climate and dirt. Similarly, Mr. Velden stated that raw material from India contained only a fraction of the international units of hCG as compared to urine collected in the Netherlands. In addition to problematizing high temperatures, he assumed that women in India would "cheat" and deliver water in order to receive gifts. The earlier question of whether poor Indian women could produce potent hCG had now been scaled up to the question of whether the country could produce pure hCG. This has to be interpreted in light of larger discursive strategies in which notions of impurity or adulteration have long been deployed by MNCs to delegitimize alternative forms of pharmaceutical production (Hayden 2013; see also Kumar 2001). In the case of hCG, the addition of fake material, poor health conditions of donors, or challenges of specific places, such as climate or dirt, were often named as factors compromising the quality of source material once collection had expanded globally (e.g., Leão and Esteves 2015, 306). Thus, evaluations of purity prevented the fulfillment of promises of economic productivity in India while simultaneously adding to the valorization of hCG in the Netherlands.

Additionally, the export of unpurified hCG might have allowed for greater flexibility regarding its final use. hCG is a volatile substance that, in its nonpurified and nonbranded state, can be turned into different kinds of end products. Organon India, for example, used to experiment with the use of crude hCG for fish breeding in Bengal (Inscape 2007). And Mothers for Mothers, the collection program in Oss, admitted that urine donated by pregnant women in the Netherlands and later in Brazil had been used to produce P.G.600, a mixture of hCG and pregnant mare serum gonadotropin that introduces estrus in pigs (Trommelen 2013). One could speculate that conducting the final purification in the Netherlands may have allowed "earlier promises embodied in things" (Tsing 2013, 23), such as the slogan "mothers for mothers," to be forgotten. In this case, processing may have created value not only by biochemically enhancing the substance but also by alienating it from its history. These attempts of erasure, however, did not always succeed fully, as the protests of Dutch women against alternative uses of their urine demonstrated (Trommelen 2013).

Remnants of Disinvestment

The commodity chain of hCG not only relied on broken promises but also reinforced global inequalities along familiar fault lines. This becomes obvious when one considers the remnants of the project a few decades later. After the Indian government began to initiate economic reforms in the late 1980s, the legal restrictions for MNCs to manufacture in India were gradually loosened. Once Organon India was freed from these obligations, the company divested the chemical factory in Kolkata. "When they got the majority [of shares]," Mr. Dasgupta remarked bitterly, "they dismantled everything we had built up." Following a larger trend of industrial decline in West Bengal, in 2003 Organon India's headquarters shifted to Mumbai, where the company once again concentrates on marketing rather than manufacturing.[23]

When the hCG production unit in Kolkata was shut down in the beginning of the 1990s, management staff was relocated within the company while low-level workers were laid off after being compensated. The relatively early closure of the hCG project was also related to the fact that a new generation of fertility drugs had been launched in the late 1980s. Recombinant hCG, which is produced using biotechnology and no longer depends on urine as raw material, was hailed in the medical world for its purity: it promised less biological contamination and more consistency in quality (e.g., Lunenfeld 2013). But while these new, recombinant versions dominate the international market today, highly purified urinary products have not lost their appeal, particularly in low-income countries. The end product is much more affordable, especially since "urinary gonadotrophins, in principle, have come off patent protection and can now be offered under generic pricing structures" (Gleicher, Vietzke, and Vidali 2003, 476). Hence, while many MNCs have shifted to only producing recombinant gonadotropins, Indian pharmaceutical companies still make urinary products, using crude hCG imported from China. And many patients in IVF hospitals in India do consume these ampoules.

The inscription on the billboard in Mr. Velden's photograph was more than a request. It also constituted a promise: the promise of fertility for childless couples that pregnant women in Kolkata could help to fulfill. Viewed in a wider context, it promised economic development for a region considered to be industrially infertile after centuries of colonial extraction. These promises mobilized a racialized, classed, and gendered set of relations on which the making of hCG as a pharmaceutical product relied. However, at a later stage, traces of these relations were obscured: they were neither detectable in the final product nor communicated in the hospital.

In the end, most promises connected to hCG production remained unfulfilled. Infertility management and population control in India, for example, took a back seat. And although inequalities between providers of bodily raw material in the global South and consumers of medicine in the global North have shifted over time, dynamics of exclusion certainly have not disappeared. Organon India not only closed down the urine collection program but also stopped manufacturing pharmaceuticals in India after economic reforms and policy changes. This is in line with more recent developments of the country's pharmaceutical sector: since the early 2000s, India does not produce sufficient bulk drugs anymore but is dependent on imports, mainly from China (Joseph and Ranganathan 2016, 11).

Nevertheless, if one asks with Anna Tsing (2015, 18), "[W]hat emerges in damaged landscapes, beyond the call of . . . promise and ruin?" one starts to note the productive side effects of Organon's presence in India. One example is a research project leading to the country's first IVF baby in the 1970s, which I describe as the second critical moment for the making of global reproductive medicine in India. At a time when India served as a provider of raw material, a doctor claimed to have produced an IVF baby in Kolkata. Yet, whereas biological material could flow rather unhindered, his knowledge claim did not circulate in any meaningful way. These processes of exclusion, on an epistemic rather than economic level, will be the subject of the next chapter.

FROM DISMISSAL TO RECOGNITION

A Contested Claim

On January 16, 2014, I attended the memorial birthday celebration for Dr. Subhas Mukherjee, who helped Dr. Chatterjee establish the urine collection scheme in Kolkata. Dr. Subhas[1] would have turned eighty-three that year. The function took place in his former flat in an upper-middle-class neighborhood in South Kolkata. As every year, Professor Sunit Mukherjee, another colleague and friend of Dr. Subhas, had organized the festivities. Around thirty people were squeezed into the small living room, where *swamis* from the Ramakrishna Mission played devotional music. Sitting on the floor and couches lining the walls, the audience faced Dr. Subhas's black-and-white photograph, carefully placed on a table and decorated with flowers. After a while, Professor Sunit got up and spoke to the guests through the microphone that had been installed for the occasion. To my embarrassment, he asked me to come "on stage" and briefly explain my research project after introducing me to the attendees with the words: "Sandra is doing a PhD on IVF in India. That is why she has to start with Subhas. Where else could she begin? She has to start with him."

The words "she has to start with Subhas" point to the ongoing controversies surrounding the beginnings of IVF in India. In this chapter, I delineate the trajectory of a claim made by Dr. Subhas about the first successful IVF experiment in India in 1978—the same year the first IVF baby had been born in the United Kingdom. Between 1978 and 2005 debates about the credibility of this claim ensued. While it was dismissed as unbelievable at first, it was recognized a few decades later among the medical community in India, although the biomedical

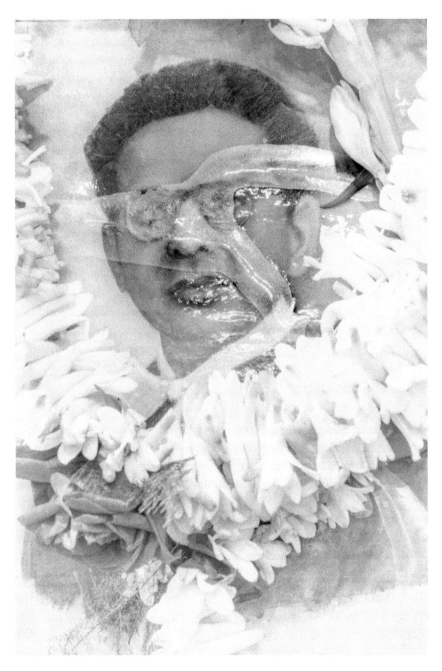

FIGURE 3. Dr. Subhas's photograph decorated with flowers at a memorial event in Kolkata. Photo by Chhandak Pradhan.

evidence itself had not changed. I argue that this rather surprising shift demonstrates the importance of space in processes of knowledge production and recognition. At a time when India functioned as a producer of raw material rather than knowledge in the field of reproductive medicine, a claim voiced from a place outside recognized centers of innovation was not taken seriously. Relying on Mary Douglas's ([1966] 2002, 36) notion of dirt as "matter out of place" and Doreen Massey's (2005, 9) relational conceptualization of space as a "simultaneity of stories-so-far," I explain the initial repudiation and subsequent acknowledgment of the claim through shifts in perceptions of legitimate spaces of innovation.

Epistemic Exclusion

It is important to note that Dr. Subhas's claim does not only affect India's IVF history. Seen from a wider angle, it "provincializes" (Chakrabarty 2000) dominant IVF historiography by highlighting the epistemic importance of the global South for the making of global reproductive medicine. More specifically, it destabilizes IVF origin stories according to which reproductive technologies emerged in the "West" and spread to the "rest." To give just one example, during the bestowal of the Nobel Prize in Physiology or Medicine 2010 on Robert G. Edwards, the responsible physiologist for the world's first IVF baby, the Nobel Prize committee noted,

> As early as the 1950s, Edwards had the vision that IVF could be useful as a treatment for infertility. He worked systematically to realize his goal, discovered important principles for human fertilization, and succeeded in accomplishing fertilization of human egg cells in test tubes (or more precisely, cell culture dishes). His efforts were finally crowned by success on July 25, 1978, when the world's first "test tube baby" was born. During the following years, Edwards and his co-workers refined IVF technology and shared it with colleagues around the world. (Nobel Assembly 2010)

The quotation is illustrative of dominant IVF historiography in several respects: the depiction of the process as a struggle undertaken by an ingenious inventor; the emphasis on "firsts," implying a focus on successful results; and the determination of the point of origin of IVF in the United Kingdom and its later spread from there. Statements echoing the latter point also surface in many scholarly accounts about the global travels of reproductive technologies.

Although scholars of science studies have long troubled unilinear modes of medical historiography by pointing to detours and contingencies, once they shifted their quite exclusive focus from science in the global North to its worldwide presence, "the dogma of its Western origins" (Raj 2013, 342), as well as concepts of diffusion, have often remained unchallenged (Prasad 2008). Bruno Latour (1986), for example, demonstrated how once facts are generated and stabilized in centers of scientific knowledge production, they can circulate quite easily in an unmodified form, a phenomenon he termed "immutable mobiles." Later on, notions of "fluid" spatialities (e.g., Law and Mol 2001) posited that the global spread of science goes hand in hand with adaptations and reconfigurations. The interplay with "local moral worlds" (Kleinman 1999; see also Inhorn 2003b) results in "vernacularized" (Simpson 2013) variants, which resonate with more general ideas about the "indigenization of modernity" (Sahlins 1999). These concepts destabilized understandings of science or biomedicine as universal and generated "empirical stud[ies] of the translocal co-production of technosciences and social orders" (Anderson 2002, 647).

Yet, although attending to creative reinterpretations conjures the agentive power of people on the receiving end of transfers (Raina 1996, 163; Raj 2013, 344), it nevertheless carries the danger of neglecting to interrogate the segmentation of the world into innovators on the one hand and imitators or reinterpreters on the other. Most accounts presuppose a point of origin located in the global North from where knowledge and technology radiate toward scientific peripheries through the centrifugal force of globalization (Prasad 2008, 37).[2] While the "West" innovates and provides the blueprint, the "rest" imitates. At best, narratives of diffusion produce the global South as an ingenious alternative to a guiding scheme epitomized by "normal" science in the global North. But they might also lead to "a cartographic exercise that designates incompliance and 'maverick' practice as localisable to the wayward developing world and good science to a predominantly Euro-American haven," as Bharadwaj (2014, 85) described for the field of stem cell research.

Departing from narratives of diffusion, Dr. Subhas's claim constitutes a proposition of simultaneity, or even anteriority, of biomedical knowledge production in the global South. Nevertheless, the controversies that unfolded after its publication also render visible the dynamics of epistemic exclusion, which prevented the claim from being acknowledged. Contrary to biological raw material, sophisticated knowledge claims could not travel easily from the global South to the North in the 1970s. However, the shift that occurred over the following decades, when Dr. Subhas's proposition turned into an established fact in India, also demonstrates that stratified topologies can morph over time.

Troubling the assumption that knowledge production only occurs in circumscribed places (mainly the laboratories of the global North; Raj 2010, 514) and taking into account the multiplication of possible spaces of innovation, also entails a rethinking of the notion of space. Narratives of diffusion rely on and promote a modernist understanding of space (in conjunction with what Dipesh Chakrabarty [2000, 8] has called a "'first in Europe and then elsewhere' structure of time"). But the "cosmology of 'only one narrative' obliterates the multiplicities, the contemporaneous heterogeneities of space. It reduces simultaneous coexistence to place in the historical queue" (Massey 2005, 5). Massey instead understands space as multiple, relational, and emergent. Her suggestion to "imagine space as a simultaneity of stories-so-far" (9) thereby emphasizing multiplicity as well as "the process of change in a phenomenon" (12), makes it possible to analyze the negotiations over India's first IVF baby as part of a shifting landscape of diverse spaces of innovation.

Contested Conceptions

In 1978, Louise Brown, the world's first IVF baby, came into the world in the United Kingdom. Only a few months later, on October 3, 1978, a television program announced that a "test-tube baby" had been born in Kolkata. The news was proclaimed by the gynecologist Dr. Saroj Kanti Bhattacharya, associate professor of gynecology and obstetrics at Calcutta Medical College, who delivered the baby by caesarian section; Sunit Mukherjee (Prof. Sunit), professor at the Department of Food Technology and Biochemical Engineering at Jadavpur University, who cryopreserved the embryos; and Dr. Subhas Mukherjee (Dr. Subhas), professor of physiology at Bankura Sammilani Medical College, the head of the operation. Dr. Subhas (1931–81) graduated in medicine at the National Medical College and completed his DPhil at Presidency College, Kolkata. A Colombo Plan scholarship facilitated his studies at the University of Edinburgh, where he earned a doctorate in reproductive endocrinology under Professor John A. Lorraine, a prominent endocrinologist who also used to be a member of the "G-Club" (Mukherjee and Lodh 2001; Chowdhury 2006). After his return to West Bengal, Dr. Subhas worked as a professor and researcher at different government institutions and ran a gynecological practice.

The pronouncement of the three researchers in 1978 was not only an assertion that they had produced the first IVF baby in India and the second worldwide. It also constituted a claim to three "firsts," since the team's approach differed substantially from the one in the United Kingdom. These were (1) ovarian stimulation with the hormones hMG and hCG, instead of conducting the procedure during an unstimulated cycle; (2) the extraction of egg cells by posterior colpotomy, instead of laparoscopic removal; and (3) cryopreservation of embryos and embryo transfer in another reproductive cycle, instead of conducting embryo transfer during the same cycle.

At first, the news was received with great interest in India: the researchers were interviewed, the condition of the baby and the mother was followed, and medical officials expressed careful enthusiasm about a possible instance of innovation. Dr. Mani Chhetri, the then director of health services (DHS), was cited in *Amrita Bazar Patrika* (*ABP*), a leading newspaper in West Bengal, as finding the claim "quite convincing. If the team could now prove it, West Bengal would get a place of pride in the medical world" (*ABP* 1978b, 1). On October 7, 1978, the three researchers were asked to submit a report to the state government of West Bengal, and they complied on October 19. Nine days later, much to their surprise, the state government's Department of Health and Family Welfare established an expert commission to examine the report "and other matters in regards to the details of Scientific principles, methodology and procedures followed for carrying out the experiments successfully" (Churchill Archives Centre, n.d.). The commission was staffed with eminent professors but without any experts in the field of reproductive biology. During a meeting with the commission on November 17, 1978, Dr. Subhas first "wanted a clarification . . . as to its legal or official status" and made clear that he and his colleagues "would not disclose the raw experimental data prior to publication in a scientific journal," as he reported later in a draft letter addressed to the DHS.[3] In another letter to the DHS on December 1, 1978, Dr. Subhas complained again about the political interference in his work by likening it to "medieval inquisitions."[4] The expert commission eventually dismissed the submitted report as "incredible" in December 1978, as *ABP* (1978h, 5) wrote: "The expert committee which submitted its four page report to State Health Minister, Mr. Nani Bhattacharjee on Saturday last, held the fact that a live human baby was born was not disputed. However, it appeared that most of the steps in the techniques adopted by the claimants for the successful transfer of 'invitro fertilised frozen thawed human embryo' resulting in the birth of a normal baby were not substantiated and with the alleged resources, the experiments referred to 'seemed unfeasible.'"

Nevertheless, the team went on to publish a short article in the *Indian Journal of Cryogenics* (Mukherjee, Mukherjee, and Bhattacharya 1978), and Dr. Subhas was able to present their findings at various conferences in India, although he was prevented from traveling abroad.[5] On January 10, 1979, the DHS proscribed Dr. Mukherjee from attending "any conference in future without prior permission from the competent authority." In another letter dated February 16, 1979, the deputy DHS specifically prohibited him to leave the country in order to participate in a meeting at Kyoto University to which he had been invited (Churchill Archives Centre, n.d.; see also Anand Kumar 1997a, 530). He was also transferred to institutions, such as the Regional Institute of Ophthalmology, that did not provide any opportunity to pursue his research interests or replicate his results

(Anand Kumar 2004, 254). Anger and pain were still apparent when Prof. Sunit recounted the reaction of his collaborator and friend during one of our meetings in Kolkata: "Subhas said after they rejected it: 'It is fine, don't believe me, I will do it again. That is how science works.' But the manner in which he was humiliated by the government, the transfer that did not allow him to carry out this work anymore . . ." According to my interlocutors, a heart attack in 1980 on top of "the humiliation he was subjected to by his colleagues in Calcutta" (Anand Kumar 1997a, 530f) led Dr. Subhas to commit suicide in his apartment on June 19, 1981.

Somatic Evidence

Before continuing the story, I want to pause to elaborate on the major points of critique that were raised against the team as well as reflect on the production of evidence in the field of reproductive medicine more generally. Prof. Sunit still wondered what it would have taken to validate their claim of innovation:

> He [Subhas] had recorded [the procedure], records were there, but there is no proof [that a baby is conceived with the help of IVF rather than naturally]. Even today, there is no proof. . . . In this last conference, this doctor [a prominent IVF clinician in Kolkata] said, "I have made two or three thousand test tube babies. And I brought some of them." So some children came on stage and performed something. But how can he prove it that these are really test tube babies? . . . I asked him, and he said, "I kept a record." But nobody has seen it besides his team. So how is that different from Subhas?

In order to prove the success of IVF, a baby is not sufficient. Researchers must not only demonstrate that they have been able to emulate the principles of a natural conception, but also make evident that they bypassed "nature," meaning that the baby has been conceived with the help of medical interventions. Dr. Subhas faced three challenges in this regard: he could present neither the baby, nor a picture of the embryo, nor evidence of the blocked tubes of the mother.

Mr. Agarwal, the father of the baby, remembered that sixteen years after their wedding, he and his wife had agreed to "try a new method" to conceive when they had consulted Dr. Subhas. While they were informed about "a chance of deformation of the baby," they were not exactly sure what the procedure entailed and did not imagine that it would create such a stir afterwards. Although one newspaper published a photo of the baby right after delivery, the parents refrained from public attention later on and were anxious to keep their daughter out of the limelight: they did not agree to give interviews to the press or testify before the government committee. "It was their duty and responsibility to have a child," Kanupriya, the now grown-up baby, explained to me, "but they did not see the need to talk about it. My parents focused on having a child, but they wanted to be left in peace afterwards. They were unambitious and they were also scared for me." They were scared that their daughter would be regarded as abnormal, as they told me, and therefore even changed her name from Durga to Kanupriya before admitting her to school. This is hardly surprising, considering that even today IVF in India often carries connotations of abnormality. It was not until 2001 that a prominent doctor who wanted to prove the team's claim (see below) managed to persuade them to sign an affidavit, which also states their reasons for reticence: "Hailing from a conservative family, we were worried of the possible repercussions to our reputation in case the child grew up to be abnormal. Our elders would not have forgiven us for having taken this step and society itself which did not know about these kinds of treatment, which are quite common today, would have scorned at our action."

In addition to the baby, Dr. Subhas was unable to present pictures of the embryo that later turned into Kanupriya. During a scientific meeting on November 18, 1978, organized by the Bengal state branch of the Indian Medical Association and the Bengal Obstetrics and Gynaecological Society at the Chittaranjan Seva Sadan College of Obstetrics and Gynaecology to discuss the team's claim, Dr. Subhas showed pictures of in vitro embryos with which he had been working earlier. "When he showed slides in the meeting, people laughed," Prof. Sunit remembered. "Someone asked, 'Is that Durga's picture?' And he replied, 'No, this was taken on another occasion.' He knew that when I handle an embryo, I should be careful with unnecessary light and handling. But people laughed. . . . Anyways, there is no proof; he could have taken the picture from a book. A sure proof would only be a genetic marker."

But even a genetic test would not have unambiguously established that the baby had been conceived through the method the team described. One doctor interviewed by *ABP* (1978a, 5) at the time got to the heart of the matter: "Even taking it for granted that the birth of the baby was effected through test-tube, there were many snags in proving it scientifically. Firstly, it was difficult to prove that the mother's fallopian tubes were blocked even before the birth of the baby. Secondly, where was the guarantee that the mother did not conceive in the natural process during the fifty-one-day period when the fertilised ovum was kept in the refrigerator before being pushed back into the mother's uterus." In this sense, the conceiving and pregnant body could not be completely trusted as a "reliable witness" (Stengers 2003, 16). In contrast to clinical realms, where natural conception is a desirable side effect, in experimental terms it constitutes a disturbing factor that has to be controlled. For this reason, later

IVF research projects only enrolled women with blocked tubes as experimental subjects, since their bodies could provide conclusive evidence that it was indeed the medical procedure that had led to conception. The critics therefore demanded another medical examination of the fallopian tubes of the mother. But the Agarwals were not prepared to partake in further examinations without any clinical benefits, as they told an *ABP* reporter at the time (1978e, 7): "'We will neither appear before the enquiry committee set up by the State Government nor will I allow my wife to be the guinea pig of the scientific community,' Mr Prabhat Kumar Agarwal, father of the baby, said in Calcutta on Sunday. . . . 'I got what I wanted. Neither myself nor my wife will take any further trouble by undergoing a troublesome medical check-up,' he added." While the Agarwals contented themselves with conception, the government committee demanded evidence of the workings of the procedure, in particular with regard to the team's assertion that it had produced several firsts. The documents provided by the three researchers were not recognized as appropriate proof for their claim of innovation—at least not in 1978.

Stabilizing IVF Histories

A few decades later, in 2002, the Indian Council of Medical Research compiled the *National Guidelines for Accreditation, Supervision and Regulation of ART Clinics* in India (a revised version was published in 2005). The guidelines included a section on the history of IVF in India that explicitly acknowledged the claim the researchers had put forth in 1978:[6] "The world's first IVF baby, Louise Brown, was born on July 25, 1978, in the UK through the efforts of Dr. Robert G Edwards and Dr. Patrick Steptoe. The world's second and India's first IVF baby, Kanupriya, alias Durga, was born 67 days later on October 3, 1978, through the efforts of Dr. Subhas Mukherjee and his two colleagues in Kolkata. . . . The techniques used by Mukherjee were markedly different from those used by Edwards and Steptoe" (Government of India 2005, 4).[7] The document continues to enumerate and recognize the team's firsts. But why did this shift happen more than two decades later? And what kind of evidence corroborated the retrofitting of India's IVF history? An attempt to answer these questions requires the introduction of two central actors: the Dr. Subhas Mukherjee Memorial Reproductive Biology Research Centre (to which I refer as the "Memorial Centre" in the remainder of this chapter) and (the late) Dr. T.C. Anand Kumar. Their interplay turned the claim advanced in 1978 into a widely accepted and officially recognized fact in India.

The Memorial Centre was established in 1985 to preserve the memory of Dr. Subhas by carrying out scientific research and convening memorial orations. Prof. Sunit, who was not only a collaborator but also a close personal friend of Dr. Subhas, was the driving force behind the foundation. He published the scientific oeuvre of his friend (Mukherjee and Lodh 2001) and organized memorial events. But all these attempts had remained relatively fruitless until Dr. Anand Kumar got involved. "All turned around after Dr. Anand Kumar. . . . Without him, Subhas is no one, he has no existence," Prof. Sunit did not tire of repeating during our conversations.

Dr. Anand Kumar was the former director of the Institute of Research in Reproduction in Mumbai and one of the leading figures of the research project that brought India's "first scientifically documented test-tube baby" into the world in 1986 (see chapter 3; Bharadwaj 2002). He received several of Prof. Sunit's invitations to memorial lectures over the years, but kept declining them, since—as he told Prof. Sunit later—his colleagues had warned him about associating himself with this group of "frauds" in Kolkata. When Prof. Sunit finally met him, he convinced him to examine the papers collected by the Memorial Centre. In the end, Dr. Anand Kumar judged them to be credible. "On going through this material, I have no doubt that Mukerji [sic] did produce a test tube baby," he wrote in one of his publications (Anand Kumar 1997a, 526).[8]

Besides publicizing his assessment in various ways, Dr. Anand Kumar managed to get Dr. Subhas's claim acknowledged by the government through the "back door." As a member of the Drafting Committee for the National Guidelines, he initiated the inclusion of the history section that mentions Dr. Subhas, according to my interlocutors. Since the document was published on a government website, the claim was not only widely distributed but also indirectly recognized by the Indian central government (Gosh 2005). Other steps followed suit, as a result of which the claim has turned into an established fact in today's medical community in India. There are conferences and symposia organized in honor of Dr. Subhas, hospital wards and research centers are named after him, doctors proudly cite their earlier association with him (e.g., Chatterjee 2011), and his name was included in a medical dictionary (Chowdhury 2006).

What is striking, however, is that the biomedical evidence has remained constant throughout this tumultuous history. It was not new insights but the report submitted by the team to the government of West Bengal in 1978 that convinced Dr. Anand Kumar, according to Prof. Sunit. But why was the claim dismissed in the 1970s and recognized in the 2000s, on the basis of the same piece of paper? Instances in which artifacts shift from fraudulent to conclusive are numerous in the history of science—a phenomenon often explained by the phrase "the time

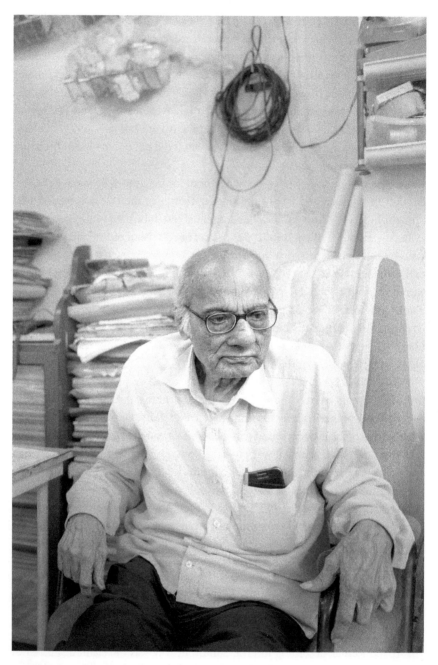

FIGURE 4. Prof. Sunit in the office of the Memorial Centre. Photo by Chhandak Pradhan.

wasn't ripe." And indeed, this is an argument invoked by Dr. Anand Kumar in one of his publications concerning Dr. Subhas (1997a, 529): the Indo-Pakistani War of 1971, the economic crisis of the 1970s, and, most important, the national state of emergency between 1975 and 1977, with its focus on population control and forced sterilizations, all resulted in a situation in which research on fertility was not met with sympathy, let alone supported by public funding. Moreover, it is probably safe to assume that a privately conducted research project on a medically elite, ethically dicey, and politically delicate topic was of no particular interest to the newly established Left Front government in West Bengal, which came to power in 1977 and was occupied with land-redistribution programs and the organization of decentralized governance structures. But the team's endeavors in the late 1970s were also an "innovation out of place," as I outline in the next section.

Innovation out of Place

Keeping in mind the notion of space as a simultaneity of stories-so-far, it is important to note that "location matters" (Abraham 2006, 217) and that the audibility of stories depends on the position from which they are uttered. "Deviation from the expected relationship between place and practice [lead] to labels of abnormality and inappropriateness" (Cresswell 2015, 190). The fact that the IVF experiments had occurred in a space that was considered out of place in several regards—outside demarcated scientific realms, outside state institutions, outside the medical community, and outside recognized centers of innovation—contributed to the dismissal of the claim.

Outside the Laboratory

When looking through newspaper reports of the time, it is striking that the procedure was unanimously termed an "experiment," thereby locating it in the realm of the laboratory (and scientific research) rather than the clinic (and medical treatment). And in contrast to the pragmatic workings of the clinic, the scientific field demands "very specific modalities of performing, witnessing and validating" (Bharadwaj 2014, 88). These modalities also entail authorized spaces where experiments can legitimately be carried out, as is illustrated by the search for the laboratory where the team in Kolkata had undertaken its research.

In 1978, the researchers were criticized for not divulging the location of their laboratory. "The committee has mentioned in its report, according to the sources, that the scientist trio have declined to disclose the location of their laboratory where they have performed the highly sophisticated job" (ABP 1978g, 7). In fact, the researchers had stated that the experiments were carried out in Dr. Subhas's flat in South Kolkata. But the thought that such a seemingly high-tech procedure could be conducted in the sphere of everyday life seemed fantastic. Even with respect to reproduction and conception—phenomena that are often associated with domestic spaces—the home appeared utterly inadequate in contrast to the bounded space of the laboratory.

Doctors opposed to Dr. Subhas's claim were skeptical because of the permeability and supposed impurity of the space, as Prof. Sunit remembered, "The doctors said, 'You did it in your home, but there must have been contamination.' Subhas said that it was better in the house. Hospitals are really dirty. And the main criterion is your own brain. Experts can do things anywhere without any sophisticated instruments. People have worked under these circumstances. Look at Pasteur: What were his facilities?" The comparison to Louis Pasteur is intriguing. According to Bruno Latour (1983), one of Pasteur's strengths was exactly his success in extending the laboratory to the field through a succession of displacements. However, he didn't start this endeavor from the home but from his laboratory at the École Normale Supérieure—a space endowed with credibility from the outset. For Dr. Subhas's opponents, the supposedly open and impure space of his home stood in stark contrast to the secluded and sanitized space of an ideal laboratory. The idea of the laboratory as a "placeless" (Kohler 2002; Livingstone 2003) space is powerful and bestows an illusion of control, and therefore credibility, regarding events happening within its borders.

The laboratory also gains legitimacy by way of social demarcation—that is, regulation of access (Shapin 1988) in terms of cultural capital, such as educational achievements or field-specific degrees. Dr. Subhas, however, chose close associates as collaborators whom he trusted and who were able to help with very specific tasks. According to an interview with *ABP* (1978c, 7), one doctor criticized this unorthodox approach by somewhat slyly characterizing the process of cryopreservation as a "miracle." He expressed doubts about the involvement of Prof. Sunit, who was not a medical doctor but a biochemist.

Outside Institutional Structures

The space of the home placed the project not only outside the laboratory but also outside recognized institutional structures. According to the Agarwals, Dr. Subhas had asked them to attend consultations at his apartment, where he was running a small clinic, after they had first visited him at his workplace in a medical college. Retreating to the home as a noninstitutional space, Dr. Subhas shielded his experiments from governmental control. He also demanded absolute discretion from his collaborators. Prof. Sunit recalled, "Subhas knew that he would have a lot of problems. He used to tell me, 'Be careful, we are holding the tail of the tiger.'" They realized that their experiments would cause a stir and might be regarded as unethical. "What if it is an abnormal child?" was a pressing question that dominated their research process, a valid one considering that IVF and cryopreservation had not yet been carried out on humans anywhere in the world. Even though the team and the parents were willing to take the risk—as Mr. Agarwal put it pointedly, "a deformed child is better than no child"—they found it advisable to retreat to the privacy of the home until they themselves could be sure about the outcome. Whereas this invisibility to state institutions made it possible to carry out the project, it later presented a challenge for the recognition of the claim.

While private clinics existed in Kolkata in the 1970s, most knowledge production was legitimized by its generation within the bounds of public institutions. This is not to say that boundary crossings did not occur. A scientist and friend of Dr. Subhas, for instance, told me about her own research on developmental embryology in a public institution, where she informally worked with fetuses that had been aborted in private hospitals. Dr. Subhas apparently received ovaries, gas, liquid nitrogen, and so forth for his private experiments either through his own appointment at a public institution or from friends employed there. Prof. Sunit also told me that the cryopreserved embryos were stored in a public facility: "The freezing was also done here in the apartment. . . . Afterwards we stored the embryos in liquid nitrogen elsewhere because it [the tank] had to be refilled. He [Subhas] had friends in labs where that was possible. Afterwards the embryos were brought back for transfer." Although government facilities were instrumental for the team's ability to carry out the project at home, the point of contention was that the researchers had announced their success from a private space without first informing the respective public institutions where they were employed. As reported by *ABP* (1978f, 8), "Dr Chhetri (the DHS) said that of the three scientists two were Government officers and 'I think they should have at least taken the permission of the Government before seeking publicity. It may be they have acted in over enthusiasm.'"

Outside Scientific Conventions

The proclamation of success through a media announcement right after the birth of the baby also sidestepped more time-consuming procedures of bestowing credibility by the scientific community, such as publication and peer review. Since the team operated outside scientific conventions and bypassed "gatekeepers of science" (Prasad 2007, 548), researchers, clinicians, and the state government could easily dismiss their claim. Even Dr. Anand Kumar commented critically on this rugged transition from concealed experimentation to public declaration. He noted that although similar controversies had emerged in the United Kingdom, a "combination of transparency, scientific debate as well as discussing moral, ethical, legal and religious issues" made the process acceptable to the general public as well as the scientific community (Anand Kumar 1997a, 530).[9]

Moreover, my interlocutors reported that Dr. Subhas was apparently disliked by senior colleagues in Kolkata, as he did not feel obliged to respect principles of seniority that are of great importance in India's hierarchical medical community. For example, he used to openly criticize a powerful gynecologist for conducting too many cesarean sections. This gynecologist turned out to be one of Dr. Subhas's fiercest critics and became the chair of the scientific meeting organized by the Indian Medical Association. Various attendees of the event reported that the meeting ended in chaos, since it was severely disrupted by senior doctors who would not allow Dr. Subhas and Prof. Sunit to present their case (see also ABP 1978e, 7). "I went to the meeting, just out of interest because I knew him [Dr. Subhas]," a scientist and colleague of Dr. Subhas detailed, "and around two hundred to three hundred people attended. Usually a paper is presented, and then there is a discussion later, but the gynecologists went there purposefully to interrupt him. They had clippings from books and shouted that he could not have done it. Finally, the meeting was cancelled." Dr. Subhas complained in a letter to the president of the association, dated November 24, 1978, that he and his colleagues had not received the allocated time to present their paper and give a demonstration of the experiment. Further, "unruly groups of people in the auditorium from the very beginning, shouting unprintable slanderous comments were allowed to continue throughout the chaotic proceedings. . . . Sir, we thought we brought global honour and prestige for the profession, and for the Country and for Calcutta, against heaviest of odds. Unfortunately, it appears to me now, that the Indian Medical Association of all organisations, was willingly or unwillingly utilized by some motivated persons to destroy that."[10]

According to Prof. Sunit, rather than being excited about a possible instance of innovation in their city, most senior gynecologists feared losing large parts of their patient load to someone who was supposedly able to perform "miracles." "He was a pioneer, and people did not like pioneers." And junior doctors "did not say anything because they were afraid that their careers would suffer." Many of my interlocutors described the interventions of Dr. Subhas's colleagues as the "crab syndrome" and as characteristic of the scientific landscape in West Bengal (see also Prasad 2005, 469).[11] They further speculated that the senior gynecologists were so influential that they were able to reverse the initial optimistic sentiments expressed by the DHS and other government officials. A contemporary politician in West Bengal who came to be entrusted with this case later on confirmed this view: "The government was under pressure by the lobby formed by his senior colleagues and transferred him where research could not be successfully pursued. . . . The doctors' community did not support him, so the government went the easy way." This was only possible because medicine and science were highly politicized spheres in India in which politicians and bureaucrats were able to interfere—in Dr. Subhas's case not only by transferring him but also by evaluating his scientific claim and preventing him from publicizing it internationally. Dr. Subhas, in contrast, was committed to an ideal of science as free from politics. According to Prof. Sunit, this attitude barred him from accepting help from politically well-connected patients and friends—a stance that made it quite unlikely that his challenge of the medical establishment would be sanctioned officially.

Outside Centers of Innovation

Finally, the project was out of place in yet another way. The claim about the successful performance of IVF in Kolkata in 1978 implied that it had not been an imitation of the technique used in England but an innovation in its own right. Moreover, the team declared that it had used different methods, thereby laying claim to several firsts. Despite the range of Bengali scientists who were highly influential worldwide during the first part of the twentieth century (take, for example, Satyendra Nath Bose, Prasanta Chandra Mahalanobis, or Meghnad Saha), the global South, much like the home, could hardly be imagined as a place of innovation in the 1970s, not only in Europe but also in India (Prasad 2014, 1).

While *ABP* reporters (1978a, 5) noted that the incident was mentioned in the British news, they also observed the "underlying tone of skepticism in the reports which will not be dispelled until the Calcutta doctors are willing to furnish further medical evidence of their achievement." Even in Kolkata, Prof. Sunit recalled, "people did not believe it could be done in India—such a sophisticated procedure which needs a lot of material." A former president of the Bengal Obstetrics and Gynaecological Society made the dimension of disbelief clear when I interviewed him in his clinic. "In those days, it was like a miracle. Without any kind of setup, only primitive equipment. This is like I would build a Mars rocket in this chamber and travel with it to Mars and back." Critics were particularly suspicious about cryopreservation, as Dr. Chakraborty, who was Dr. Subhas's senior colleague, told me. "It was not acceptable at that time. Especially cryopreservation had not been done in humans. It was not known. And then people thought one needed electricity for that, and Calcutta was known for its power cuts."

Complaints about such "constraints of location" (Prasad 2014, 86) were omnipresent. And it is not to deny that infrastructural challenges were certainly pronounced at that time. Many doctors told me that even in the 1980s and early

1990s, they had to smuggle much of the equipment required for IVF to India when they went on conference trips abroad. Prof. Sunit reported that Dr. Subhas had to spend a lot of his salary on maintaining his laboratory. Further, some of his well-off patients supported him in procuring materials abroad, and he sometimes received pharmaceutical samples from Organon India in exchange for advisory services. Many clinicians also pointed out that clinical procedures were not highly sophisticated or rigorously standardized at that time. Dr. Chakraborty, for instance, described practices in Kolkata during the 1970s and 1980s as "uncivilized" to me. He provided the example of monitoring the surge of luteinizing hormone before ovulation by a—in his opinion "very crude"—procedure that often resulted in lost egg cells. "Every two hours, urine had to be taken at night. We did this like tribal people, but now everything is civilized." These widespread "colonialist discourses" (Traweek 1992) of scientific underdevelopment made the production of a "high-tech baby" in Kolkata in 1978 highly improbable.

Dr. Subhas, however, defended himself by emphasizing that it was not the equipment that was central but the expertise and skills he had acquired through earlier experimental work in this field. In an undated, typed-out interview he states, "Durga is not a miracle child, but the fruit of long-term research and systematic and scientific study. I have successfully conducted experiments on about a hundred rats and mice though surprisingly it wasn't successful on monkeys" (Churchill Archives Centre, n.d.). Prof. Sunit also remembered, "Subhas always said that IVF requires high skill, not so much the instruments. Freezing is not complicated; [freezing] cow semen, you can do it in a cattle shed. What is complicated is the synchronization with the uterus [to estimate an opportune time for embryo transfer]. . . . The DHS also asked us, 'How do you know when to transfer, there are so many hormones?' But Subhas just used to see the cervical fluid and its viscosity: 'If it is sticky like a gum, it [the embryo] will stick.' There were three transferred, and one stuck." Another example mentioned by Prof. Sunit is the incubator in which Dr. Subhas stored early-stage embryos. In contrast to contemporary incubators, it enabled the researchers to control only the temperature but not the mixture of gases inside the device. Dr. Subhas therefore used to take out the vessels containing embryos once in a while and blow on them in order to provide the necessary carbon dioxide. A commentator in *ABP* argued at that time that it is exactly these instances of lack that encourage an attitude of inventiveness:

> That despite the absence of delicate and sophisticated equipment the team had the daring to conceive and carry out such an experiment is indeed admirable and offers an eloquent commentary on the capability and resourcefulness of India's medical men and scientists. In fact, the

lack of experimental facilities was a test for the ingenuity of the doctors who were ultimately obliged to adopt methods distinctly different from those followed in Britain. . . . Since all the details of the long process through which Calcutta's test tube baby was born is yet to be made public, it is too early to visualize the possible impact which the achievement will make on the various branches of science. (*ABP* 1978d, 6)

As demonstrated, the impact remained minimal even though colleagues of Dr. Subhas, like Dr. Chakraborty, were inspired to continue his work after his death in order to "prove that it is not impossible in our country" (see chapter 3). But in 1978, India remained confined to a space of imitation in the scientific landscape; a space that innovations diffuse to rather than emerge from.

Shifting Topologies

Place matters when innovations have to stand the test of credibility. The Kolkata team's claim was dismissed because the researchers were not able to make themselves heard, owing to their "offside" position. They conducted and revealed their experiments outside legitimate spaces, such as the sterile laboratory, the public institution, the rule-obeying scientific community, and the well-resourced research environment. As Dr. Subhas's home in Kolkata was out of place in several regards, it could not lend credence to a claim of innovation.

Although imagined geographies of legitimate spaces of innovation proved to be consequential, space is also "mobile and mutable" (Livingstone 2003, 8). More than two decades later, the transformation of the team's report from an insufficient document to a sign of proof became possible through the advocacy work of the Memorial Centre and Dr. Anand Kumar. Moreover, a generational change in the medical and political fields in Kolkata, a shift away from the exclusive focus on population control in family planning programs, the flourishing of the IVF industry in India, and the establishment of IVF as a normalized and standardized medical procedure that had long lost its connotation of being something out of the ordinary (see chapter 3) all contributed to the reevaluation of the claim in the late 1990s and early 2000s.

Furthermore, it was reassessed in a different spatial constellation. In addition to a greater acknowledgment of India's political and economic standing by the global North, the country's self-conception as a scientific superpower—take for example the nuclear and space programs—contributed to a reconfiguration of the landscape of legitimate spaces of innovation. India could now be imagined as a place in which novelties originate. This was certainly facilitated by a growing interest in fostering scientific innovation, coupled with the promotion and valuation of "indigenous" technology by the central government during the 1990s and 2000s (e.g., Government of India 2003; see also Abraham 2000, 167).[12] Guidelines and policies eventually cumulated in the declaration of 2010–20 as the "Decade of Innovations" by the then prime minister, Manmohan Singh, at the Inauguration of the 97th Indian Science Congress (Government of India 2010). Dr. Subhas's story—as an epitome of "indigenous" ingenuity—fits this agenda nicely and can now be called on to promote India as a pioneer in IVF, a locus of medical expertise, and a powerful player in a globalized medical market (e.g., Tikku 2013).

Similar to the global South, noninstitutional and domestic spaces were also reclassified as potentially innovative places. Take for example the mythos of "garage inventions" so popular in the entrepreneurial world in the United States, which now translated more easily to India and its growing knowledge economy (e.g., the IT sector); or later, the rise of citizen science and do-it-yourself laboratories that purposefully circumvented institutional structures, which resonated with the widespread praise of *jugāṛ* in India, a concept of bricolage that productively combines lack and inventiveness. These changes became palpable in stories of second-generation researchers in India, who started IVF in the 1980s. They could proudly proclaim that they began their IVF career in unpropitious spaces, such as garages or storerooms, improvising "with locally available materials."[13] This is not to say that power differentials have completely dissolved (for a vivid example, see Bharadwaj 2014). But even though established centers of innovation do remain influential in many respects, global asymmetries prove to be dynamic (Raina 2003), and the spaces in which claims of innovation can be reasonably put forth have grown larger.

Prof. Sunit's recurrent insistence that the history of IVF in India has to start with Dr. Subhas attests to the fact that the acceptance of the claim still stands on shaky ground. Throughout his life, Prof. Sunit therefore continued to fight for Dr. Subhas's definite recognition by both the state and the central government. From the disappearance of the history section in the Assisted Reproductive Technology (Regulation) Bill, one may assume that the central government was unwilling to take the risk of formally sanctioning the claim and, consequently, disrupting dominant IVF historiography, which credits the first cryopreservation and the first ovarian stimulation to Australia and the United States, respectively. And although the Kolkata team's work has been widely acknowledged in medical circles in India, it remains largely unnoticed on a global level.

The trajectory of Dr. Subhas's claim is nevertheless remarkable. Over several decades, it shifted from an incredible proposition in the 1970s into an established fact among medical circles in India two decades later. Imagined geographies of innovation combined with "technoscientific Othering" (McNeil 2005, 109) prevented the claim from being acknowledged at first, as it was voiced from a space considered to be out of place. One of the reasons that made its retrospective recognition plausible was altering topologies of scientific and biomedical power—from central institutions in the global North to decentralized spots in different parts of the world. Simultaneity was now more readily conceivable, at least for my interlocutors in India. The fact that the country's IVF sector also got fundamentally reshaped over the following decades certainly helped Dr. Subhas's case. For reasons that are the subject of the next chapter, India could now be imagined as a place that innovations emerge from rather than diffuse to.

FROM HOBBY TO INDUSTRY
How IVF Diversified

On a pleasant afternoon, I met Dr. Indira Hinduja in her well-established private hospital in one of Mumbai's affluent neighborhoods. She was part of the team that had produced India's first "scientifically documented test-tube baby," born on August 6, 1986. The project was headed by Dr. Anand Kumar, then director of the Institute of Research in Reproduction (IRR) who later publicized Dr. Subhas's claim. In addition to the IRR, the public King Edward Memorial (KEM) Hospital took part in the project. Located in Parel, a former working-class neighborhood in Mumbai that used to house employees of the city's textile mills, KEM Hospital opened its doors in 1926. A few hundred meters from its colonial structure, hustled into a small lane, stands the modern building of the IRR (today the National Institute for Research in Reproductive Health). Founded under the Directorate of Family Planning of the Government of India in 1954, from 1963 onward the institute has been governed by the Indian Council of Medical Research and entered into a partnership with KEM Hospital to "conduct application-oriented research" (National Institute for Research in Reproductive Health, n.d.). Further, the IRR's initial focus on family planning has broadened over the years, particularly since the "beginning of the twenty-first century when the institute decided to adopt [a] more holistic approach towards reproductive health" (National Institute for Research in Reproductive Health, n.d.).

During the 1980s, Dr. Hinduja was associated with both public institutions: she worked as a gynecologist at KEM Hospital and also became a PhD student at IRR. She remembered how she had to organize her scientific work around clinical duties in the hospital while conducting research on IVF: "Pickups [egg cell

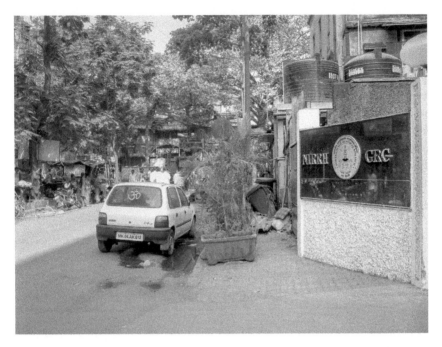

FIGURE 5. Entrance to the National Institute for Research in Reproductive Health with a view toward KEM Hospital. Photo by the author.

retrievals for IVF] used to be done [in the operation theater of KEM hospital] before the working hours in the mornings at five or six o'clock. Because at eight o'clock, the routine care starts. And we have to give away the [operation] theater . . . then carry [the egg cells] to the laboratory [in the IRR], keep them in place, come [back to the hospital] at eight for the routine work. Then during lunch time, go [to the lab] and do the fertilization, and after four the entire lab work had to be done, preparation of the media, exchange of media." Although her double appointment translated into long hours and a constant back-and-forth between the clinic and the lab for Dr. Hinduja, the institutional collaboration also proved to be advantageous: the large patient load of the hospital made recruiting experimental subjects easy and provided access to biological material. However, a few years after the experiments had turned out to be successful, the IVF program at KEM Hospital was discontinued. Some of the involved researchers went on to establish private clinics. And it took almost twenty years until another public IVF unit would open its doors in India.

This account of IVF practice in the 1980s as an exceptional research endeavor, jointly conducted by two public institutions, stands in stark contrast to contemporary circumstances where I interviewed Dr. Hinduja in her private hospital, which handles IVF as a routine medical intervention. It shows how IVF has transformed: from an experimental "hobby"—as Dr. Chakraborty called it—into not only a standardized medical procedure but also a profitable product offered by mainly private providers. After describing experiments by second-generation researchers in Mumbai and Kolkata in the 1980s that led to India's first scientifically documented test-tube baby, I examine the routinization and commercialization of IVF over the 1990s—processes that were closely related to the country's economic reforms. The concomitant transnational flows of medical supplies and financial investments not only led to the flourishing of India's IVF industry but also contributed to the emergence of a global fertility market since the 2000s. I then provide a detailed analysis of the formation of a diverse and uneven field of medical providers in Delhi and situate the city's contemporary institutional landscape within the context of India's postcolonial health care policies. Changes in terms of processes of privatization and corporatization as they have become prevalent over the past decades do not constitute clear-cut ruptures, however: public hospitals, for instance, have offered IVF in Delhi since the 2000s. This is but one example of how the public and the private blend into each other and culminate in a highly diverse IVF landscape, resulting in stratified treatment options and unequal access to services.

Improvised Interventions

In the 1980s, two main research projects followed Dr. Subhas's footsteps, and both of them succeeded with their IVF experiments in 1986. In addition to the publicly funded project in Mumbai, one colleague and one student of Dr. Subhas in Kolkata—Dr. Chakraborty and Dr. Sudarsan Ghosh Dastidar—continued his work on a private basis. Similar to Dr. Hinduja, both of them used to earn their living as gynecologists while conducting research. In contrast to today, "IVF provided no income," Dr. Chakraborty explained. "I took it as my luxury, a hobby. I started to do something new. To get a good name." Eventually, his plan proved to be successful. Between 1986 and 2019 Dr. Chakraborty used to head a well-known, private fertility institute in Kolkata.[1] Today, IVF constitutes not only a medically standardized but also an economically profitable procedure.

The following section focuses on narratives of physicians and embryologists who were involved in IVF research in India during the 1980s and early 1990s. These pioneering projects resemble each other in terms of their experimentality on the one hand and their integration into daily clinical life on the other. Slightly similar to Adriana Petryna's (2011) account of the ways in which clinical trials have become normalized as a form of health care delivery in some parts of the world, experimentality used to be part and parcel of everyday clinical life in India during this time. Most IVF research was conducted in gynecological clinics. Or, to put it differently, most IVF procedures in hospitals or nursing homes constituted improvised interventions (for improvisation in medical practice see Livingstone 2012; Street 2014).[2]

Improvisation permeated clinical life in various ways. As shown earlier, notions of lack in terms of material infrastructure dominated the narratives of clinical pioneers. However, in contrast to Dr. Subhas, to whom this lack proved to be detrimental during the recognition process, the second generation of IVF researchers in India could present themselves as risk takers who were able to overcome adverse circumstances in creative ways. Pointing to the garage adjacent to his old clinic, in which he started his IVF career, Dr. Chakraborty proudly referred to it as a "cowshed." Instances of lack and improvisation were also prominent in Dr. Hinduja's account. Even though the team in Mumbai started its research in 1982, the first baby was delivered only in 1986. "In the absence of previous experiences with embryological and surgical procedures, it was not until 1985 that a full-fledged IVF-ET program could be launched," an explanation by the Indian Council of Medical Research (2000) reads. Dr. Hinduja detailed how the team had to overcome various hurdles during these years: "incubator would not work, electricity would go off, somebody will not come, fertilization did not occur, we didn't even know where the water comes from. . . . So, we kept on changing, that is why it took a little longer. We used to change everything, we used to sit and discuss what can it be, if fertilization did not happen." In this way, improvisation constituted an integral part of clinical life for many IVF pioneers before standardized protocols took over.

A similar sense of improvisation prevailed in terms of training. There were no formal educational institutions offering degrees related to IVF in India in the 1980s. Clinical pioneers mainly relied on short visits to laboratories abroad and conversations with researchers there. The team of the IRR, for example, visited Jones Institute in Norfolk in 1985 with funding provided by the World Health Organization (Anand Kumar 1997b, 15). Other doctors consulted academic journals: "My infertility teachers were journals. . . . *Human Reproduction*, which came from Europe, and *Fertility and Sterility*, which came from the US. I used to read every article on IVF, read the methodology, and then convert it into practice. So my true teachers were *Fertility and Sterility* . . . mainly *Fertility and Sterility*. And through that, it was like self-training, putting into practice what I read in books and in the journals. . . . The real teachers were these journals."

While journals provided theoretical instructions, practical experience could only be gained through actual interventions. Doctors thus acquired and trained their skills by way of clinical practice. "Everything was by hit and trial," explained one physician. "People from different branches entered [the profession] and they just tried various things. There was no formal training, there was no degree, there was no certification of any kind. . . . Everything was pure experimentation." Similarly for embryologists: although some of them could draw on experiences with animals, most tried IVF on humans without any specialized training.[3] One embryologist, who used to work with animal gametes before she started human IVF, told me, "It was on an experimental basis, I was not sure whether I would be successful. . . . I was given the chance to try on humans without any training. But animal and human are identical to some extent. . . . I used common sense and it worked." Thus, although IVF developed within established gynecological clinics, it simultaneously constituted a highly experimental procedure. Or, as one clinician put it, IVF developed in the form of "research-cum-service providing."

As elsewhere in the world, people who had no other hope of conceiving decided to submit themselves to these improvised interventions. The mother of the first scientifically documented test-tube baby in 1986 was a twenty-three-year old local schoolteacher and wife of a municipal corporation worker in Mumbai. After news of the IVF pregnancy had been publicized, couples from different regions and of various backgrounds started to approach KEM Hospital, as a newspaper report from that time documents: "They have come from Dubai, London, Vellore, Chitraput, Hyderabad, Delhi and the suburbs of Bombay, on an anxious pilgrimage to the KEM Hospital. Most of them are in their mid-thirties; a few are forty. . . . Today, over fifteen new patients arrive at her [Dr. Hinduja's] clinic every morning, some straight from the railway station. She gets a similar number of letters every day . . . from all over the country" (Jain 1986). This report suggests that (international) travel for IVF has a long history. Even Dr. Subhas received letters from abroad as early as the late 1970s inquiring about the possibility of undertaking IVF in India. A couple who described themselves as "Indian from Hindu Family settled in USA for fifteen years" wrote to him on February 24, 1979: "We felt that the above news [the birth of the test-tube baby] came as God's message to us. We are married for the past fourteen years and do not have a child since my wife had undergone an ovarian cyst operation and one of her ovary was taken out. One of the American Doctors has advised us to go to either India or England to have a test tube baby. Since we feel that we will be comfortable with Indian Doctors, we decided to come to India for this purpose." Their doctor in the United States had advised them to go abroad, as "it cannot be done in this country because of strict AMA [American Medical Association] rules." Thus, since the late 1970s, hopeful patients, often with protracted histories of infertility, were ready to travel long distances to undergo an experimental procedure.

Dr. Ghosh Dastidar acknowledged the help of his former patients decades later when he dedicated a "lifetime achievement award" that he received at a conference in Delhi to them. As he explained to me after the bestowal of the award,

> That is why today I dedicated to the patients. . . . Now I know in 1982, 1983, 1984 I did a lot of mistakes. And I did a lot of, not harm, lot of trials you can say. Not guinea pig [trials] but trials on patients because IVF came directly as a clinical procedure without being properly tried with proper clinical trials. . . . Because the demand was so high. Once Louise Brown was born it came to flood the world. Many centers, even not knowing very well how to deal with embryos, they started IVF centers. Not only in India, in many parts of the world. Those patients we must acknowledge their support. They came forward and that's why we know so much today.

While IVF research in India had become possible with the help of a diverse group of patients who agreed to undergo clinical experiments, once the procedure had been proven to work, the clientele became more homogeneous. The collaboration between the IRR and KEM Hospital in Mumbai, for instance, continued after the first successful case, as the research team had to reproduce their results. In 1988, Anand Kumar et al. reported that 121 patients had undergone IVF in the hospital, resulting in seven live births and one ongoing pregnancy at that time. However, once Dr. Anand Kumar retired in the early 1990s, funding from the IRR stopped. This meant that IVF was not available to patients in KEM Hospital anymore. As Dr. Hinduja stated, "We developed the technique, they [the IRR] published the data, they redocumented it, they reproduced it, so they are not going to continue. It is research, not service-oriented. And because it costs a lot of money, they did not want to continue that. To produce one baby if it costs so much, you might as well treat other conditions like tuberculosis, diarrhea. It is very true. We have developed it, disseminated the knowledge, and then other people started. That is how I left the hospital and started a private practice." Dr. Hinduja and Dr. Anand Kumar both continued to practice in the private sector, switching to a for-profit model. This resembles developments in other parts of the world: Robert G. Edwards, for example, described how he and his colleagues planned to scale up IVF in the United Kingdom after their successful experiments. However, "[n]o governmental support was forthcoming, so our work was halted for 2.5 years after Louise Brown's birth. Finally, venture capital was obtained, and Bourn Hall [a private hospital] opened" (2001, 1093). Only the provision of private capital enabled IVF's routine clinical application. Similarly, once IVF in India had become like a "textbook treatment," as Dr. Hinduja put it, government support dwindled.

Further, the procedure turned into a viable and even economically productive option for clinicians and other investors. Today, "in every corner, there is IVF," Dr. Hinduja continued. "Everybody is doing well. Why not? There is a lot of requirement for that. The success rate is good, everything is fine, so more and more people should take advantage of it." What Dr. Hinduja omitted from her account, however, is that patients who have been able to take advantage of the text-book version of IVF are people who can afford to pay for it. While patients at KEM Hospital used to contribute around 1,500 to 2,000 Rs. for pharmaceuticals and tests, the cost for IVF in the private sector was estimated to be as high as 50,000 Rs. at that time (Jain 1986). And it has increased ever since. By the late 1990s, IVF had morphed from an experimental project into a standardized, profitable product that was mostly accessible to the country's upper-middle classes. In this sense, IVF's transformation "from frontier to mundane" (Wahlberg 2018, 12) in India went hand in hand with its commercialization (Bharadwaj 2016, 119).

Medical Supplies

In a timely coincidence, the routinization of IVF overlapped with the country's economic reforms and its concomitant changes in trade regulations. Since the mid-1990s, medical distributor companies have provided the material infra-structure necessary to conduct IVF as a standardized and commercialized procedure. They have made the pharmaceuticals, disposables, and technical equipment required for IVF easily available to clinicians. One could thus argue that the economic reforms provided the conditions of possibility for the immense growth of India's IVF industry in the 1990s and 2000s. Moreover, new opportunities of foreign direct investment coupled with a legislative void provided the financial and legal base to turn India into a global fertility market.

Many clinicians mentioned that before the 1990s, imports of medical equipment proved to be complicated and costly because of protective trade regulations and high import duties. "It was difficult to procure all the stuff that you needed in the lab in India," said one doctor. "Everything, whenever I'd go out on a trip, I'd bring stuff or I'd ask my friends to bring it in." Other clinicians manufactured tools on their own, such as pipettes or even incubators, and mixed their own media—the fluid in which gametes and embryos are cultured. As one embryologist recalled, "The formula for media was not given in the literature. Since I was in research I kept trying, and if it was not good, I threw it. Media was simply tested on some eggs and sperm, mostly sperm, because . . . of [its] availability. If sperm survives, then the egg also survives. I used to make my own media for fifteen years."

The reduction of import duties in the 1990s allowed medical distributors to successfully sell ready-made media as well as other equipment produced outside India to IVF practitioners, often in cooperation with foreign partner firms.[4] Dinesh, the owner of the first IVF distributor company in India, stumbled upon this opportunity in 1993. He was working as a service manager for laboratory equipment, when a clinician asked him to procure culture media for her. When he started to import ready-made media from a Danish company, business was slow at first: most doctors were wary about the media's quality, fearing that the cold chain might have been interrupted during import procedures (see also Bharadwaj 2016). And indeed, Dinesh often had to destroy media that got held up in customs and turned out to be unusable. He remembered that senior clinicians "were not even willing to try it. But then it happened—not with the high client people, but I contacted the young aspiring people: 'You try this.' . . . The cold chain was a big challenge. I personally used to travel by train and carry it in thermos. Those were the times. People realized it gives good results and it is very convenient, it makes your life easier. . . . Senior doctors realized it very late. Now 99 percent [of clinicians] use ready-made media." Junior clinicians' increasing interest in IVF provided Dinesh with clients who had neither the experience nor the patience to manufacture media on their own. Conversely, his supplies further contributed to the growth of the IVF sector by simplifying the procedure and publicizing it among doctors. One could argue that the rising number of IVF clinics in India and the growing market for IVF equipment were mutually dependent and cross-fertilized each other. Today, the equipment industry remains powerful in the IVF world and "competes with the pharmaceutical industry as a major player in shaping medical opinion" (Nagral 2012, 11). Distributor companies not only design and furnish whole IVF units according to specific budgets, but they also provide training and clinical support to doctors and embryologists.

Layered Landscapes

The current IVF landscape in India is often depicted as a dynamic industry and global marketplace. While this is certainly an adequate characterization, what is frequently omitted from this representation is the diversity and stratification of this landscape: There exist different kinds of institutions, and IVF is practiced in heterogeneous ways. Below, I describe the formation and differentiation of Delhi's institutional IVF landscape in detail. Delhi constitutes an interesting case because a variety of providers have been offering their services in the city: from charitable hospitals to for-profit nursing homes to corporate hospitals to public facilities. This diversity is closely connected to India's broader history of health care policy since Independence.

Private Entrepreneurs

After the birth of Delhi's first IVF baby in Sir Ganga Ram Hospital in 1991, private facilities—sometimes in the form of charitable hospitals but mainly in the form of for-profit nursing homes led by entrepreneurial doctors—have been dominating the city's institutional IVF landscape. While the exclusive presence of private IVF institutions in the 1990s and early 2000s was certainly due to the state's reluctance to engage in further research, it also reflects more general developments of the privatization of health care in postcolonial India. In 2005, Sengupta and Nundy explained that "[w]hen India became independent of British rule in 1947 the private health sector provided only 5–10 percent of total patient care. Today it accounts for 82 percent of outpatient visits [and] 58 percent of inpatient expenditure" (2005, 1158). These numbers are indicative of an immense growth of the private sector over the past decades.

In response to the report of the Bhore Committee of 1946, postcolonial health policy at first focused on the expansion of primary health care through public institutions.[5] But starting as early as the late 1960s, the privatization of health services turned into a political priority (Baru 2001, 211). "Due to global recession, this process received a boost during the late seventies and early eighties, enveloping both developed and developing countries, imposing fiscal constraints on government budgets and encouraging them to cut back on public expenditure in the social sectors. This increased the space for the growth of the private sector in the provisioning of health care, which was accelerated during the eighties and nineties with the increasing role of the pharmaceutical and medical equipment industries in seeking markets for their products" (Baru 2006, 2). The National Health Policy of 1982 specifically emphasized the importance of private providers to contribute to the goal "Health for All" (Burns 2014, 91). The shift toward privatization was further corroborated by the propagation of structural adjustment programs and economic reforms. This coincided with the time when entrepreneurial doctors, like Dr. Nishika, started to establish private, for-profit IVF hospitals.

Dr. Nishika[6] is a well-known and respected IVF specialist in Delhi, and during my fieldwork she owned and ran her own hospital—PremiumIVF. PremiumIVF is located in one of the upper-class residential areas in South Delhi, close to major traffic junctures and yet shielded from the busy streets by lush trees. The three-story building used to be a family residence and still exudes a homely atmosphere. Red and white sun blinds greet visitors approaching the center, and cool air surrounds them upon entering the space. To reach the reception desk, patients cross a waiting room lined with leather couches. The interior design conveys an understated elegance, with medical awards and baby pictures decorating the rooms. Always busy, PremiumIVF is mostly frequented by upper-middle-class patients. However, the remnants of a charity program for people from lower socioeconomic backgrounds are still visible—although its size has clearly diminished since government centers have opened IVF units in Delhi. Upon entering the consultation room, many patients are captured by Dr. Nishika's aura. Calm and confident, she receives patients sitting behind an impressive wooden desk. Dr. Nishika started her career in 1983 as a gynecologist, after she had completed her medical training in India. One day, a TV program about IVF caught her attention: "I was watching one of the news channels, and I think Louise Brown had just been born—it was a few years after that. There was this program on TV where they had shown the entire development of the embryo and things like that, and how the whole process took place. So, I think I was extremely fascinated and I thought that's what I should focus on, rather than general gynecology." In 1993, Dr. Nishika decided to enroll in one of the world's first taught master's degree programs on reproductive biology in the United Kingdom. In addition to studying embryology, she also attended clinical consultations. Upon her return to India in the mid-1990s, she started to practice IVF in her own hospital. Since her IVF patient load has grown steadily, she eventually decided to give up all other gynecological and obstetrical work in 2000 in order to concentrate only on infertility.

As there were hardly any embryologists in India, Dr. Nishika conducted the laboratory work on her own until she met Dr. Shila, a PhD in biochemistry, whom she trained and still employed during the time of my fieldwork. Many of the clinical entrepreneurs I talked to emphasized that they are potentially able to do all IVF-related work on their own. As another director of a nursing home mentioned, "You have to develop yourself as a multidisciplinary person. You have to develop all the disciplines in yourself. I am trained in everything now, and I am not dependent on anyone." They claimed to know the whole procedure by heart—a status that would set them apart from novices in the field. "Most IVF is like an elephant and four blind men," another clinician explained. "Someone is doing the ultrasound, someone the embryo transfer, someone is counseling, and someone is doing the hormones. All is done by someone else and everybody talks about different things. I do all of it together." While a few doctors still rely only on their own expertise, most clinicians eventually started to employ other specialists, such as embryologists or radiologists. The division of medical labor has further intensified with the establishment of corporate hospitals.

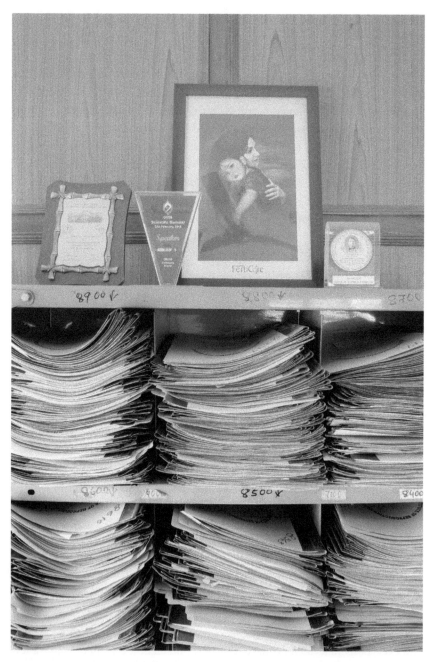

FIGURE 6. Patient files and medical awards in an IVF hospital. Photo by Chhandak Pradhan.

During my fieldwork, Dr. Nishika started to work part-time as the director of a newly established IVF unit in an Indian-owned corporate hospital. While she appreciated the specialized care corporate hospitals can offer, she always remained critical of their "commercial approach," as she put it. A few years later, however, she eventually gave up her own nursing home after she (together with other Indian IVF specialists) started to collaborate with a European hospital chain. PremiumIVF was dismantled and, once again, turned into living quarters. The trajectory of Dr. Nishika's professional career reflects a wider shift in Delhi's IVF landscape where clinical entrepreneurs now compete with large-scale corporate hospitals, sometimes backed by international capital.

Corporate Competition

Starting from the mid-1980s, novel financial mechanisms have radically transformed private health care in India. In 1986, the hospital sector was recognized as an industry, "which meant that financing was available from public financial institutions" (Thomas and Krishnan 2010, 2). Furthermore, "[i]n the 1990s, big business houses started to float shares in the market for the hospitals they set up" (Sujatha 2014, 256). With the Indian government's repeal of restrictions on foreign direct investment in the hospital sector in 2000, the private health care sector further turned into an investment opportunity for global capital. This implies that apart from the earlier described quantitative changes, qualitative differences have manifested themselves.

> The private sector has been the dominant provider of healthcare services [since Independence], but the pattern of private participation has changed considerably. . . . In the first phase, private participation mostly comprised practitioners providing primary and secondary care through individual clinics. The second phase was marked by the rise of small hospitals (less than 30 beds), owned and managed by doctor entrepreneurs, providing secondary care, mainly in urban and affluent rural areas. The last decade has seen private capital flowing more into establishing large tertiary care hospitals (more than 100 beds) and corporate hospital chains. (Srinivasan and Chandwani 2014, 1508)

Alongside charitable hospitals and clinical entrepreneurs running their own nursing homes, the contemporary IVF landscape in India is now dotted with corporate hospitals, which are mainly multispecialty, tertiary care institutions. In Delhi, the first corporate hospital was established in 1996 (Hodges 2013b). As private, for-profit hospitals, corporate hospitals "differ from other nursing homes in their private corporate limited status" (Lefebvre 2008, 88). The Indian state explicitly provided support to them through tax exemptions as well as the "provision of land, water and electricity at lower cost, and concessions on import duty on diagnostic equipment. The only condition was that [corporate hospitals] should provide 30 percent in-patient facilities and 40 percent of the out-patient/diagnostic services free of cost for people below poverty line" (Qadeer and Reddy 2006, 8; see also Lefebvre 2008), an agreement that is hardly ever respected (Public Accounts Committee 2005; see also Lefebvre 2010, 24).

The utilization of corporate hospitals has clearly been an upper-middle-class experience. Waiting times are short, and hospitality standards high—a reason why corporate hospitals are frequently compared with five-star hotels. "The[ir] premises, with their display of prosperity, wealth and modernity, enable patients to assert their difference and identity" (Lefebvre 2008, 99). More recently, corporate hospitals have also started to cater to an international clientele, advertising their services in various countries. Appealing to foreign customers with "first world health care at third world prices" (Turner 2007), corporate hospitals—supported by the Indian state—strive to turn the country into a global medical market.[7] In 2004, the government even "declared that medical treatment of foreign patients is legally an export and eligible for all fiscal incentives extended to export earnings" (Deomampo 2016, 43).

Most corporate hospitals in Delhi have added IVF units to their range of medical departments. Whereas these represent competition for already established practitioners, for gynecologists who do not own nursing homes or who try to expand their practice, they may provide favorable job opportunities or even stepping-stones to self-employment. There are different "doctor engagement models" utilized by corporate hospitals, ranging from treating clinicians as full-time employees with fixed working hours and salary, to renting spaces to doctors and collecting a certain fee per case from them, as well as mixed models (Bakshi and Burns 2014, 158–59). Doctors working in corporate hospitals often voiced concerns in conversations with me about directives from hospital management to aggressively recruit new patients, conduct a fixed number of procedures, or grow revenues in other ways (see also Sama Resource Group for Women and Health 2010). This "entrepreneurial spirit" (Nagral 2012, 10; for a more general description of an "enterprise culture in neoliberal India," see Gooptu 2013) has significant consequences for the manner in which clinicians can exert their profession. The practice of "target-oriented medicine" is aggravated by the fact that until today the private IVF sector has remained largely unregulated.

When I met Dr. Aishwa, she used to work for an Indian-owned corporate hospital. She had received her medical degrees from prestigious medical colleges and universities in Delhi. After living in the United Kingdom for the past few years, where she had practiced as a gynecologist and infertility specialist, Dr. Aishwa decided to return to India and started working for a corporate hospital. Since she was still struggling to establish her "patient base," her colleagues regularly advised her on how to "increase her numbers." They suggested to "create awareness" about infertility by acting as an expert in media appearances (for the media/medicine nexus, see Bharadwaj 2000) or by organizing welfare camps in the areas surrounding the hospital. Conducting camps allows physicians to identify potential patients, attract them with cheap initial tests, and publicize the hospital's infertility unit (Sarojini, Marwah, and Shenoi 2011). Another suggestion was to organize a continuous medical education event or a conference for gynecologists who could later refer IVF patients to her. Conferences often entail practical training sessions for rather simple procedures, like IUI, in the hope that junior doctors later refer the more complicated (and revenue-generating) cases to specialized hospitals. Dr. Aishwa's struggle made apparent that the rising number of IVF units in Delhi has resulted in a situation where clinics compete over patients. Bharadwaj (2016, 232–35) similarly notices that IVF centers in the 1990s were not always financially viable. Physicians are therefore expected not only to provide medical services but also to create demand for them. This is exacerbated by the fact that Delhi's IVF landscape remains highly diverse: charitable hospitals and entrepreneurial nursing homes are still standing their ground, while the public sector has entered the stage again.[8]

The Return of the Public Sector

Since the 2000s, the IVF landscape in Delhi has further diversified through the establishment of publicly funded IVF units—a development that Kate Hampshire and Bob Simpson (2015) have called "assisted reproductive technologies in the third phase," a phase during which IVF becomes more affordable and accessible for larger parts of the population. Out of the three government hospitals in India that offered IVF during the time of my fieldwork, two were located in highly specialized research and teaching institutions in the city. Additionally, one of the IVF units run by the Indian army was based in Delhi.

The return of the public sector has to be read in the light of larger developments over the 1990s and 2000s, such as the global conceptual shift to include infertility in reproductive health programs as heralded by the United Nations International Conference on Population and Development in 1994 or the growing understanding of health care as a right in India, for instance through several Supreme Court rulings. However, since the Indian state spends only about 1 to 1.5 percent of its GDP on health care (Burns, Srinivasan, and Vaidya 2014; Widge and Cleland 2009), and fertility management does not constitute a political priority, the establishment of high-cost IVF units could not have been realized without the efforts of committed doctors.

A former army officer and gynecologist, who established the Indian army's first IVF center, recounted how he mobilized support from various groups: "When my seniors saw my enthusiasm, they gave me some sum for a research project. But it was not much, just three lakhs [300,000 Rs.]. And an incubator was already five lakhs [500,000 Rs.]. So, the industry also helped, they let me pay the incubator in installments." Along with the medical industry, his future patients contributed to this endeavor as well. "There was a British-era labor room which I cleaned with the help of my patients. If you put in 100 percent, then only the system starts helping you. I did not wait for funds or facilities, but with the help of the patients we cleaned and sanitized this building." This story is similar to the ones I heard about the establishment of the two public IVF units in Delhi located in well-known research and teaching institutions. Doctors contributed a high amount of personal effort by persuading bureaucrats about the importance of IVF as well as mobilizing their own political connections. The director of the IVF unit where I conducted my fieldwork, which I call CommonCare in this book, had struggled for years to upgrade the fertility services on offer in the hospital. Dr. Sumitra recounted how an IVF unit had always been her dream since she joined the attached medical college in the 1980s as faculty: "It took so long. First, I had to convince people, my administrator, that we really need the IVF center. Because population of India is so much, they cannot think that some group of patients requires IVF also. So, I finally convinced them, and the center started. It took long." Earlier she had to refer patients to the private sector, whenever her sparse resources were exhausted, knowing all too well that most of them could not afford it. Dr. Sumitra and her colleagues were finally granted a space in the hospital that they remodeled according to their needs.

Today, their IVF unit caters to a diverse group of patients. Most of them enter CommonCare in much more convoluted ways than the straightforward path in PremiumIVF. Patients at CommonCare do not even set foot in the IVF unit during their initial appointments. Rather, they visit the busy infertility outpatient department, where physicians examine them and record their medical histories. Patients are then advised to conduct diagnostic tests at various other departments so that clinicians can determine whether they qualify for IVF. Once they have accomplished all these steps (which can easily take a couple of weeks or months) and have successfully been identified as IVF patients, they are admitted to the unit. Entering the IVF unit, patients have to register at the reception desk early in the morning. After that, they begin their wait in the space next to the reception, the walls decorated with posters explaining the "miracles of conception." Because of the senior doctors' other duties, patients often have to spend several hours waiting, not knowing when they will eventually have their turn (for waiting and IVF, see Bärnreuther 2019).

While general treatments in public hospitals are supposed to be completely free, patients undergoing IVF in the two units in Delhi have to contribute financially by either paying a lump sum or purchasing their own pharmaceuticals. And in case some services are unavailable because of shortage of resources, patients also have to raise money for that. Only low-income workers covered through the Employees' State Insurance Scheme or government employees covered through the Central Government Health Scheme receive a reimbursement of their expenses later on.[9] Even if patients have private insurance, providers in India do not pay for IVF. Particularly the high charges for the pharmaceuticals used during ovarian stimulation (to grow more than one egg cell) prove to be a financial burden for many IVF aspirants.

Some doctors therefore try to find low-cost solutions to make IVF more accessible (for low-cost IVF, see Ombelet 2007). Employing medical protocols that require fewer or no pharmaceuticals, they reduce the cost of ovarian stimulation to a considerable extent. Further, physicians also use cheaper drugs, such as urinary instead of recombinant gonadotropins. The urinary hCG that is currently produced in India (see chapter 1) is regularly deployed in government hospitals. Finally, some doctors try to reduce the prices of drugs by negotiating discounts with pharmaceutical companies. Others buy pharmaceuticals in bulk and then club patients into "batches" or share supplies with colleagues. Dr. Sumitra, for instance, mentioned that she is able to reduce the costs for ovarian stimulation by a third (from around 60,000 Rs. to around 20,000 Rs.). When medical procedures are adjusted to patients' financial abilities, the stratification of Delhi's IVF landscape manifests itself not only in terms of access but also through medical practice.

Cross-Fertilizations

Although private and public hospitals practice IVF in distinct ways by catering to distinct clienteles and providing distinct kinds of care, it is important to note that the private sector itself is extremely diverse and that low-cost private clinics often have more in common with well-equipped government units than five-star corporate hospitals. Moreover, the public and private are not clearly demarcated realms. As illustrated, the successful workings of government projects often depend on connections with the private sector. Without the help of medical distributors, the army officer could not have bought his first incubator. And Dr. Sumitra gives many patients access to the IVF unit in CommonCare because of the discounts she has negotiated with pharmaceutical companies. Private companies, in turn, profit from the government sector because of its large sales numbers.

Conversely, the private sector heavily relies on public resources: not only in terms of generous incentives for corporate hospitals but also in terms of degree programs in public medical colleges that bring forth a new generation of gynecologists. Many doctors described an "ideal" career path as moving from a public hospital, where they receive extensive training, to private and more specialized centers, where salaries are higher (Baru 2000).[10] After learning their trade and refining their skills on a diverse and undemanding patient population, many clinicians proceed to more profitable grounds.

Patients as well switch between public and private realms: for example, every time certain tests were not available at CommonCare, they had to procure them from private laboratories. There were also few patients who had first consulted private practitioners but eventually ended up in CommonCare either because they had run out of money or because they wanted to undergo more expensive diagnostic tests for free, and then again change to a private setup for the actual IVF procedure. Thus, boundaries between the public and private sectors prove to be porous, allowing clinicians and patients to navigate this landscape in flexible yet stratified ways.

The comparison of Dr. Hinduja's account of the experiments in Mumbai during the 1980s with her medical practice today makes apparent that processes of routinization and commercialization considerably changed IVF practice in India over the past decades. When IVF pioneers started to conduct experiments in the 1980s, there were no training programs in place, doctors had to gain experience by way of improvisation, and a reliable material infrastructure still had to be established. The fact that the beginnings of India's IVF sector coincided with the country's economic reforms enabled the industry to grow. The provision of pharmaceuticals, disposables, and technical equipment through medical distributors facilitated the transformation of IVF from an experimental hobby to a standardized procedure and profitable product. These shifts also went hand in hand with the privatization and corporatization of India's health care sector more generally. Today, the country's IVF landscape is often depicted as a transnational marketplace, although the second half of this chapter has painted a more nuanced picture of its institutional diversification in Delhi.

Attending to the diversity of Delhi's IVF institutions challenges "bland clichés about the 'third world hospital'" (Street 2014, 34) on the one hand and "shining India" on the other. From charitable hospitals to for-profit nursing homes to corporate hospitals to public facilities—the city's IVF landscape remains layered to this day. IVF's embeddedness in various institutional cultures and constraints implies that the procedure is not performed in a stable and homogeneous manner. Rather, IVF practice has been shifting over time and continues to oscillate between an exclusive high-cost intervention and a low-cost alternative. In the following chapters, I analyze IVF's contemporary making in Delhi in more detail. In doing so, I shift registers from the relations that have shaped reproductive medicine to those that it generates in contemporary practice.

THE CLINIC AND BEYOND

Reproductive Temporalities

It is not uncommon to spot statistics in IVF hospitals in Delhi that posit rather unrealistic success rates for IVF cycles.[1] A few clinics even display them prominently in waiting rooms. A sign in one private hospital, for example, stated, "IVF Success Rates: 1st cycle: 40%, 2nd cycle: 70%, 3rd cycle: 90%." Proclamations of success nourish hope (Franklin 1997), particularly if people encounter IVF after a long and exhaustive trajectory. In these cases, IVF often appears as a "last resort" to create "own" offspring. IVF promises not only conception (for the "quest for conception," see Inhorn 1994) but also the establishment of genealogical relations through the couple's "own" reproductive substances. What other scholars have observed with regard to surrogacy is thus true for IVF more generally: it enables "many infertile couples to 'chase the blood tie' (Ragoné 1996) in pursuit of biogenetically related offspring" (Deomampo 2016, 7).

In this context it is important to note that reproductive substances are not "mere physiological substances of reproduction but meaningful social endowments of ancestral and affinal identities and potencies" (Sahlins 2013, 65). To put it in other words, gametes carry relational potential beyond biogenetic meanings. Catherine Waldby (2019, 9), for example, describes how Australian women understand egg cells to be "eminently relational, linking women back into their family history, laterally into their relationships with husbands and partners, and forward into their relationships with children, actual or potential." Although egg cells are sometimes understood to connect past, present, and future in similar ways in IVF clinics in North India, sperm counts as a more powerful relational

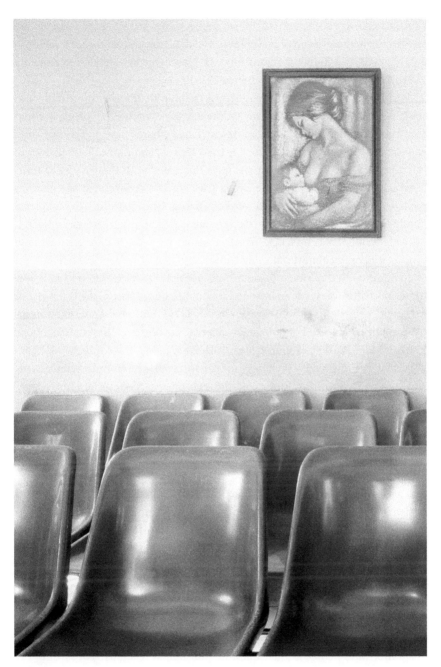

FIGURE 7. Waiting room in an IVF hospital. Photo by Chhandak Pradhan.

substance. In predominant patrilineal perceptions, genealogical relations are created through the bond of male blood, which is transmitted through semen—a condensed and highly precious form of blood (for Sri Lanka, see Simpson 2004b; see also Copeman and Banerjee 2019).

In this chapter, I follow IVF patients in Delhi in their quest to establish substantial relations over time. Relying on the narratives of five IVF patients whom I have gotten to know well during my research and whom I have met several times at different stages of their reproductive trajectories, I show how their relations to infertility and medical interventions have fluctuated with the passage of time. Most patients described their treatment trajectories as convoluted and onerous paths (*rāstā*). Rather than narratives of progress from infertility to completed family, "'negative' temporalities of delay or failure" (Abram and Weszkalnys 2011, 14) were prominent experiences. The five narratives evolve in different ways with distinct outcomes, almost reflecting clinical statistics of success and failure.[2]

In addition to describing patients'—often cyclical—relationship to IVF over time, the chapter serves as an introduction to the clinical part of the IVF process, in which further dimensions of temporality come into play. Describing mundane medical practice, I observe how patients "flow through the clinic" (Inhorn 2015, 26) and IVF cycles unfold over time. Andrea Whittaker (2015, 131) suggests that IVF hospitals constitute liminal spaces where "time is reorganized" and "bodily rhythms [are] regulated through pharmaceuticals and hormones." Although medical interventions are indeed designed to hormonally manipulate bodily rhythms in order to make (particularly female) bodies productive, I also show how clinical practice attunes to somatic time. Clinicians, patients, technologies, and pharmaceuticals make IVF work—not only by working *on* but also by working *with* bodies.

The chapter thus weaves together various reproductive temporalities connected to IVF: the linear quest of patients to continue genealogical relations through reproductive substances; the cyclical relationship to IVF characterized by setbacks and new trials; and the calibration of time in IVF hospitals when bodily rhythms are regulated on the one hand and medical interventions are ordered around bodily temporalities on the other.

Stagnation

What motivates people in their quest for substantial relations? For most of my interlocutors, parenthood "equal[ed] normalcy" (Becker 2000, 1) and constituted a crucial "next step" in a couple's married life. "It is very important to have a child, that is the second thing after marriage that people expect from you," remarked one woman. Not being able to take this step was experienced as a severe "reproductive disruption" (Inhorn 2007; see also Franklin 1997), often described in terms of stagnation. "It is time to move on," "we wanted something new in our life," or "I am ready to step into motherhood" were common statements articulated by my interlocutors. The husband of an IVF patient even invoked the four stages of the Hindu life cycle. In doing so, he located himself at the transition to the stage of a householder (*gṛhastha*)—a stage he was eager to embark on.

But infertility does not only put a couple's life on hold. It may also threaten the future of a lineage. Many patients understood it as their duty to bear offspring (see also Bharadwaj 2016). Especially newlywed women reported that they feel a moral responsibility to "give a baby" and, even better, a son to their new household, as marriage is seen to serve the prime purpose of continuing the patrilineage (*vaṃś āge baṛhāne ke lie*) (Singh 2017).[3] Many interlocutors pointed out that "you get married in order to continue the patrilineage [*vaṃś*], that is doing your duty [*dharma*]." One's "own" reproductive substances, particularly semen, are of prime importance in this regard.

Additionally, some women spoke about their wish to experience pregnancy and childbearing at least once in their lifetime. I met postmenopausal patients who had already adopted a child but still tried IVF with a donor embryo in order to be able to give birth and regain their sense of womanhood. "It should be one time that I give birth, one time," explained one of them. The ability of IVF to extend reproductive time after menopause (with donor eggs or donor embryos) did not allow her to give up. As one clinician remarked, "Now a lot of older people are coming. Previously older people did not use to bother. They thought if they cannot have, they cannot have." The relatively high numbers of postmenopausal patients is related to the understanding of infertility not only as a medical but also as a moral condition. Nonconception might turn men into useless (*bekār*) husbands and, more often, women into barren (*bānjh*) wives. Women occasionally reported that they confront situations where they are not allowed to attend community functions or are shunned by neighbors and relatives because of their infertility (for descriptions of cultural conceptions of infertility and the attached stigma, see Patel 1994; Unnithan 2010; Bharadwaj 2016).

While reproductive technologies lengthen the time frame during which women are expected to bear children, the medicalization of infertility through reproductive medicine may also relieve them from blame by turning a moral concern into a medical condition. Upon entering the clinic, infertility turns into a disease that can be diagnosed and potentially cured. Especially the routinization of semen analysis helped to shift structures of blame from women experiencing the sole responsibility of childlessness toward at least considering the possibility that the "fault" might lie with the husband. While, as many doctors recounted, a few years ago many men were not even willing to provide a semen sample for medical analysis, it has since turned into a routine procedure. And in cases in which semen quantity or quality were defined as below average, dynamics between couples often changed. One doctor even employed the strategy to never explicitly state that the semen is "good" in order to avoid the "blame game." While I have seen both partners expressing feelings of inadequacy or insecurity when the medical diagnosis indicated their "fault," only women ever voiced the fear of grave consequences, such as divorce and the husband's remarriage (see also Inhorn 1996). Puja, a patient I met in CommonCare, had faced these threats from her mother-in-law.

Puja

As she visibly enjoyed telling, Puja had met her husband under adventurous cir-
cumstances. It was a "love marriage" that her mother-in-law had opposed from the
beginning. Puja, a teacher and beautician, was too educated for her mother-in-law's
taste—she would have preferred a "village girl." Hence, trouble was foreseeable, but
her mother-in-law's harassment intensified when no offspring was in sight—a par-
ticularly urgent issue for the family, as Puja's husband is the eldest son. Luckily for
Puja, her husband could not be convinced to remarry. "My mother-in-law told my
husband to leave me and get married again but my husband refused." Later on, she
urged Puja to do whatever it took to give birth to a grandchild. "She told me that
there were so many different procedures to get pregnant, and I should pick one of
them." Seven years later, after nothing had worked, the mother-in-law threw Puja
and her husband out of the house.

I met Puja in the tiny home that she and her husband had built in a poor
neighborhood in the far west of Delhi. She had already undergone one unsuccess-
ful IVF cycle in CommonCare and was currently contemplating another. Even
though her husband would rather leave this topic once and for all, Puja was now
consumed by it.

> He says that I should not bother for all this, and there are people who live
> without kids. But at the end of the day, women have this feeling in their
> heart to have a baby of their own. . . . My husband tells me to leave all
> this but I am sure I will get him to agree. We just built this house so we
> are low on cash these days. . . . We have some loans to pay off, but once
> they are done . . .

Puja believed that she would be able to arrange the sum she would need for a second
IVF cycle through her participation in a women's self-help group. The women in
the organization support each other by providing a certain amount of money every

month to assist one of them with a project (for an example of raising money for IVF with bingo events, see Roberts 2012, 74).

As Puja's story demonstrates, it is not only the obligation to produce offspring that makes people mobilize large financial resources. Long after the family had already broken up over the issue, Puja still tried to conceive. Other patients I talked to also expressed a strong desire to have children in order to overcome feelings of absence and loneliness. Children were considered to "complete" the couple and "make life meaningful" (Bärnreuther 2019). They wished to care for someone and have "something to look forward to" when returning from work, like Neha, whom I will introduce in more detail later on:

> I come home and there is nothing to look forward to except cook food, cook dinner, and go to bed. Get up in the morning and go to work. So it is that thing that is missing. Bringing up a child, helping him with his studies. There is nothing to look forward to. First you are looking forward to getting married, then you get married. Then you look forward to having another change in your life, which is your children. Then you grow with your children. In our lives we have nothing to do. All we look forward to is switching jobs or planning a vacation but then we are lonely at the end of our day. Although we are happy with each other. He [Neha's husband] is quite happy, he doesn't miss anything in life, he does not feel any void, but I do feel that.

Reproduction proved to be important in several respects for my interlocutors: it may provide a family with offspring and continue the family line, but it may also mean the fulfillment of a personal desire and constitute an important step in a couple's relationship. "Reproduction involves many actors and competing pulls of duty, desire, and care" (Singh 2017, 24). Social expectations, familial demands, and personal desires are often inextricably entangled, and all conglomerate in the need to have one's "own" child. To Puja and Neha, childlessness presented itself as a condemnation to stagnation within their lives, relationships, and families (for the United States, see Becker 1994; for the United Kingdom, see Franklin 1997). But rather than considering alternative means of reproduction, such as adoption (Bharadwaj 2003), both pursued their quest for substantial relations through medical interventions.

The Right Time

Infertility is recognized as a medical condition by the World Health Organization (WHO) and, among other factors, it is defined temporally. The clinical description developed in 2009 characterizes infertility as "a disease of the reproductive system defined by the failure to achieve a clinical pregnancy after 12 months or more of regular unprotected sexual intercourse" (Zegers-Hochschild et al. 2009, 1522). Or, in another WHO document (2010), infertility is defined as "the inability of a sexually active, non-contracepting couple to achieve pregnancy in one year." Besides the inability to conceive, the common basis of both definitions is the time span of twelve months. Infertility, hence, stands out from other medical conditions in that it is characterized not only by specific symptoms but by its duration over a certain period of time.

The temporal dimension mentioned in the WHO definitions incidentally overlaps with the point of time when many couples in India start to experience their reproductive life as problematic and consider consulting specialists. Interlocutors reported that if there was no "happy news" between a few months and two years after their marriage, they would undertake "first steps." During my research, I only met couples who identified as married, and, if not otherwise indicated by patients, doctors took the wedding as the starting point of their efforts to conceive. Couples who used contraceptive methods after their marriage counted the time from the moment when they started "trying for a child."

The right time to seek medical interventions is determined not only by the amount of time that has elapsed since starting to "try" but also by the amount of "social pressure" people face. My interlocutors described social pressure as manifesting itself either openly by manner of exclusion and stigmatization or in more subtle ways, for example in the form of suggestions to "do something"—whether conducting rituals (*pūjā*), visiting auspicious places, or consulting doctors. Pressure may prompt couples to undertake a higher number of interventions or start with procedures earlier than initially intended. For example, a couple I met in PremiumIVF had decided to not immediately undergo an IVF cycle after learning about the wife's blocked tubes. They had planned to first enjoy their time alone together and focus on their careers. But pressure from their family eventually led them to pre-pone their IVF cycle: "We are not in a hurry . . . But in India you are pushed into parenthood as soon as you get married because of familial and social pressure. We don't have any issues [to wait] but it is custom," the husband justified their decision.

As well as constituting an element that drives patients into doctors' chambers, time serves as a major criterion in medical decision-making processes. When new patients arrived in the consultation room, and doctors noted down their reproductive history, the first questions they posed were, "How long have you been married?" and "Since how long have you been trying for a child?" In doing so, they established whether the medical definition of infertility applied and what kinds of interventions were justified. When recently married couples visited the clinic, doctors would send them home with the instruction to try for a few more months.[4] Natural conception, they explained, is not an easy process and it might require a few months till "it clicks." Couples who turned up after a few years of childlessness, however, were often reprimanded for coming in "so late."

Another temporal factor that figures prominently in medical decision-making is the age of the female patient. In biomedical understanding, female bodies possess only a certain number of egg cells that are eventually exhausted over the course of a woman's reproductive life (Martin 1987). The age of the female patient thus determines the urgency of interventions. Yet the so-called chronological age of a patient does not necessarily overlap with her gynecological age—that is, the state of her ovarian reserve. Hormonal and other tests are therefore employed as "time planners." They are understood to trace the progressive decline of fertility and aid in decisions about whether and how soon IVF should be undertaken. In order to determine appropriate medical procedures, doctors thus employ various temporal measurements: the time since the couple started trying for a child, the chronological age of the female patient, and her gynecological age. These constitute guidelines for diagnosis as well as the appropriate progression of interventions.

Not all patients visiting IVF clinics receive a definite medical diagnosis (e.g., blocked ovarian tubes). Oftentimes their state is labeled "unexplained infertility."[5] In cases where routine diagnostic procedures yield no results and the underlying reasons of infertility remain unclear, doctors suggest trying a specific order of interventions. In these cases, suitable fertility management is conceived of as a process of trial and error that ideally unfolds at an appropriate speed. After conducting initial tests and monitoring cycles, doctors might start with stimulated cycles (i.e., only prescribing hormones for ovarian stimulation). Later, they might conduct IUIs before advising patients to undergo IVF.[6] In this scheme, IVF itself may eventually serve as a means of diagnosis (Franklin 1997, 146), as it may expose otherwise hidden flaws, such as bad egg quality or dysfunctional fertilization. The temporal relation between diagnosis and treatment is inversed in these cases, as diagnosis happens retrospectively as part of the treatment regime. Or, as Gay Becker (2000, 16) puts it, "the proliferation of assisted reproductive technologies has led to a paradigm shift in which infertility care is driven not by the diagnosis, but by the treatment."

There are rules of thumb about how many cycles of a particular intervention one would try in a row; after five to six unsuccessful cycles of IUI, most doctors suggest patients to "move on" to IVF. Yet the "right" point in time is not easy to determine: patients and doctors have to walk the fine line between progressing to possibly unnecessary, invasive, and expensive interventions too soon, and losing time by proceeding too slowly—or "wasting time in being conservative," as one doctor put it (for the United States, see Becker 2000, 17). Many patients felt that they had lost precious time during earlier stages of their treatment trajectories (see also Whittaker 2015, 105). When they eventually were advised to use IVF, many decided to take their chance.

Treatment Rhythms

An IVF treatment cycle unfolds in specific rhythms. It starts with ovarian stimulation, a procedure during which clinicians administer hormonal pharmaceuticals to female patients in order to achieve the growth of several follicles that contain egg cells. While this stage of the cycle is designed to hormonally manipulate the female body in order to make it productive, clinical practice also attunes to bodily rhythms. For example, ovarian stimulation can only start on day two or three after the onset of menstruation. In case patients visit the clinic at other points of time, doctors ask them to return on day two of the next cycle. In this sense, the body's monthly reproductive cycle predetermines the time frame within which medical procedures can be conducted.

One strategy to bypass the specific rhythms of patients' bodies is the "down-regulation" or "suppression" of their menstrual cycles with oral contraceptives. Downregulation turns the reproductive body into a "clean slate," as doctors call it, which can then be manipulated according to clinical schedules by adding hormones. This method is used when clinicians conduct IVF in a "batch system," where the reproductive cycles of various patients have to by synchronized.[7] This is necessary if hospitals employ freelancing embryologists who are available only for a couple of days per month, so that egg cell retrievals and embryo transfers of all patients have to happen on the same day.[8] Yet many doctors criticize the batch system as not taking into account peculiarities of individual bodies, as Dr. Isha, a junior doctor in PremiumIVF, explained. "Sometimes the hormones rise early and then the patients ask, 'Why don't we do it [the retrieval] now?' So what to tell them?" Hence, even if bodies can be refashioned in ways that are convenient to clinicians, they might not deviate entirely from their idiosyncratic rhythms—a fact that clinicians have to adapt to and work with.

At times, patients request doctors to start their IVF cycle within a specific time frame (e.g., in a particular month or after a certain date), according to advice from astrologers. As one patient explained, "We do things parallel, we do not only rely on one method. Celestial bodies influence your fate. My mother-in-law asked an astrologer, according to the birth charts. He told us that in September and October there is a good time for trying, so we thought it would be a good opportunity to do IVF now." Besides that, more down-to-earth concerns are taken into consideration as well: one day when Dr. Isha was in the middle of determining the approximate timing for an IVF cycle, the patient suddenly interrupted her calculations. "Actually, could we move it to next month? I don't want the child's birthday to be in the summer . . . it's too hot for birthday parties." When starting the ovarian stimulation process, doctors thus have to calibrate different temporal logics relevant in IVF clinics (Thompson 2005, 9–10): bodily processes, clinical schedules, astral configurations, or even future birthday parties.

During ovarian stimulation, hormonal pharmaceuticals are administered to patients on a daily basis through injections. Their impact on patients' ovaries is overseen by vaginal ultrasound examinations, which are the primary means in a complex regime of monitoring to capture the so-called "response" of bodies.[9] When patients enter the darkened ultrasound room and hurriedly undress in one corner, the doctors assembled flip through their medical files. As soon as the preparations are completed, and the patient's body is placed on the couch where the scans take place, it has entered "clinical territorium" (Heimerl 2013, 72), meaning it becomes available for clinical inspection. After the insertion of the ultrasound probe, the clinicians' eyes immediately turn to the glimmering screen of the scanner conveying a constantly shifting black and white image. For patients, the screen is invisible, as it is placed behind their head. And in contrast to prenatal scans, during which doctors sometimes provide elaborate explanations, patients are usually ignored during monitoring sessions. This is corroborated by their behavior: most of them distance themselves from the goings-on in the room by remaining silent, looking at the ceiling, or closing their eyes (78). Eventually, a picture of the reproductive tract appears on the screen, in which follicles, which contain egg cells, are discernable as dark circles. Once a segment of the ovaries that encompasses most of the growing follicles is brought into focus, the image is frozen. This provides clinicians with the possibility of measuring the diameters of follicles by plotting a line across the black structure in the picture. The numbers that appear on the computer screen are noted down on monitoring charts. They enable comparative assessments over time and are used to determine the pace of follicular growth. These results, in turn, elicit specific instructions from physicians. Based on these figures, clinicians take decisions about dose adjustment, which they briefly communicate to patients, simultaneously noting down their instructions in medical records.

If a patient's body responds well to the pharmaceuticals, which means a gradual growth of multiple follicles, the dosage continues. In case follicles grow in a pace considered to be too fast or too slow, the pharmaceutical regime is adjusted accordingly. Thus, although the female body is manipulated and monitored through pharmaceuticals and technologies, the body's response simultaneously dictates medical interventions. Many doctors therefore consider IVF not only as a set of practices shaping bodies but also as a process during which they have to pay careful attention to them. At the same time as they fashion bodies, doctors listen to them. "Let's see what your body says," or "it depends on the response of your body," were frequent comments uttered in hospitals. Hence, while patients themselves remain quite silent during the time of ovarian stimulation—some authors even argue that they become "collaborators" in their medicalization (Whittaker 2015, 107; see also Thompson 2005)—their bodies turn into responsive entities, engaging with and contributing to biomedical practice.

Just to be clear: bodies do *not* adhere to a communicational model of signal-response (Martin 1987, 40), which suggests that pharmaceutical input according to fixed protocols is directly translated into a certain somatic output. In CommonCare, for example, clinicians were always pressed to explain to the central supply agency that they simply cannot determine the required amount of hormonal pharmaceuticals, as it varies between bodies. While there surely are clinicians who employ standardized stimulation protocols, most of the doctors I worked with disdained this approach. Years of experience enabled them to relate to every body in distinct ways: they carefully listened to and were in turn responsive to patients' bodies in a constant modulating process of finding the right dose that results in the right response. For example, when Dr. Nishika started working for a corporate hospital in which protocols were standardized, she refused to use the fixed doses suggested by the management of the hospital. "Every patient is different," she explained. "It is not just a technique where you are just doing something without evaluating, without thinking. Every couple is an individual couple rather than a factory setting. You cannot conduct this like an assembly line." She therefore continued to design ovarian stimulation protocols customized for particular patients' bodies. This constant back-and-forth between clinical manipulation and somatic response surpasses simple mechanisms of stimulus-response, as responsive bodies constantly demand creative adaptations from physicians. During ovarian stimulation, doctors thus work not only *on* but also *with* bodies in order to turn them into productive entities.

In cases in which clinicians encounter bodies that are not responsive, medical procedures are discontinued. For example, in case a body does not respond to ovarian stimulation in a productive way, all procedures are stopped and a rhetoric of stagnation (e.g., "sleeping ovaries") and even lifelessness is employed, reflecting prevailing concepts of infertility as an unproductive state (Martin 1987). "It is of no use to beat a dead horse," was Dr. Isha's answer to a situation when a treatment cycle had to be abandoned because a patient's body had not presented itself as responsive. She made it clear that it is not in the clinician's power to change these situations: "We can only work with what nature has provided us. . . . If there are no eggs, you cannot bring them up." Thus, only those bodies that exhibit sufficient and adequate growth of follicles in terms of quantity and pace are valued as being capable of undergoing assisted reproduction.[10]

Once follicles reach a certain size, patients receive a "trigger" shot of hCG to finalize maturation. Roughly thirty-six hours later, just prior to the expected time of ovulation, egg retrieval is scheduled. At the same day when eggs are extracted from the woman's body during a small surgical procedure, her partner "collects" semen in the hospital. The prepared egg and sperm cells are then fertilized in the lab either in a petri dish (IVF) or through micromanipulation (ICSI). A few days later, the resulting embryos are transferred to the uterus during a procedure that resembles a pelvic exam. Exactly two weeks after embryo transfer, a pregnancy test is conducted. These stages of the IVF cycle constitute a predefined sequence, almost a treatment rhythm with which patients become familiar. "I am very comfortable with the cycle, I know what's going to happen, I know what to expect," said Neha after her fourth IVF cycle. Time, in this scheme, is highly structured: it is expressed in segments of months, days, or hours and can be visualized on calendars in a linear way.

While this form of clocked time prevails as a hegemonic mode of temporal measurement in the clinic, it is rather unhelpful in expressing patients' experiences of an IVF cycle. Duration between treatment events is not necessarily perceived in terms of equal time bits; rather, time may stretch or contract (Serres 1998, 60). While some phases of IVF cycles may pass by very quickly, others may appear endless. The most poignant example for the experience of stretched time are the two weeks between embryo transfer and pregnancy test, a time of high anxiety about whether implantation has occurred or not. While the IVF process before embryo transfer is characterized by constant monitoring, these two weeks are defined by ambiguity. The state of the embryos transferred to the uterus cannot be visualized by ultrasound or hormonal tests, since they do not produce any meaningful traces yet. As one patient explained, "Beyond the transfer there is nothing that can be monitored for two weeks. You can feel changes inside, sometimes there are cramps and you just don't know what is happening. I wish they would come up with some monitoring process during this time." Since clinicians cannot elicit medically intelligible data during these two weeks, every patient is treated as potentially pregnant: the medications continue, and they are only stopped if the pregnancy test turns out negative. Many patients corroborate these measures with their own precautions: when returning from the embryo transfer in the operation theater to the recovery room, they move slowly, swaying from one foot to the other and holding their abdomen to prevent the embryos from "falling." Some also take leave from their jobs, avoid abortive food, and spend the time till the pregnancy test resting at their mother's house, like many pregnant women in North India who return to their natal home (for similar precautions in Thailand, see Whittaker 2015, 117). This period of waiting seems to last forever and plays an incisive role for the experience of IVF cycles as exceptional.

In general, IVF represents an experience out of ordinary time for many couples. It puts routine life on hold (Becker 2000, 176; Franklin 1997, 168) and reschedules daily activities. "Now it is work that revolves around doctors' appointments, not the other way round," remarked one patient. Many people even quit their jobs or took leaves: "I quit my job, because I thought that it will add to the stress and I can be more concentrated on that [IVF]. And it is difficult with office: you have to wait for hours [in the hospital], then you have to go upstairs to get injections, it takes a whole day. And you have to do frequent visits." For most patients medical interventions become a priority in their lives for a couple of months or even years (Bärnreuther 2019). However, when IVF cycles are successful, normality is regained soon after. In the twelfth week of pregnancy, most IVF centers transfer their patients to a "normal" obstetric department in a "normal" hospital where delivery will take place.[11] Many patients are thus able to normalize their exceptional experiences in retrospect. As the brother of an IVF patient put it once his sister's baby had been born: "Now it is yours, it is not IVF anymore." But when IVF cycles remain without positive results, different dynamics unfold.

Setbacks

Although, numerically, failure constitutes the norm, patients whose pregnancy tests turn out to be negative experience the lack of success as a severe setback. They often described surprise and disappointment when they realized that their body has failed them once again. "There was so much emptiness, frustration, so much waste," said a patient whose IVF cycle had failed earlier. "Now I don't consider it anymore as the end of my life," she continued. "It cannot be an endless journey. It is not in my hands. But this feeling of sorrow is always going to be there." Amita, as well, had to cope with disappointment not only because her IVF cycle had failed but also because her body had only produced a low number of egg cells.

Amita

When I met Amita and Vivek in PremiumIVF in 2012, they were very hopeful that their current IVF cycle would work out. It was the day of their egg cell retrieval, and in the morning they had stopped at a temple to receive blessings for the procedure. Doctors and IVF can only help to a certain extent, they said, everything else is in god's hands.

After their arranged marriage four years ago, Amita followed Vivek to the United States—the country where he had studied and then worked as an engineer. When they returned to India one year after their marriage, people immediately started to ask questions about their reproductive status. They therefore decided to consult a doctor: first, Amita had several cysts removed from her uterus, and then they tried IUIs for a while. Since nothing happened, their gynecologist eventually referred them to PremiumIVF. During our first encounter Amita had already told me that she experienced IVF as an exhaustive and invasive procedure. This was related to the fact that her ovarian reserve turned out to be low, and that she had to endure an exceptionally long time of ovarian stimulation.

As I found out during our second meeting, their pregnancy test had been negative. Amita was shocked about the result, which she perceived as a double failure: not only the IVF cycle but also the ovarian stimulation had not been very successful. "I could produce only three eggs, despite all the assistance and the medication. There is nothing wrong with my husband. One [egg cell] was not healthy, one was [grade] A and one was [grade] B. They transferred these [last] two. We trusted them and did not question anything." Especially since she had put so much trust in her doctors, Amita was disappointed about the clinicians' indifference when the cycle failed. "Doctors were very indifferent. I would just have needed a pat on the back, nothing big. I did not even get to see the senior doctor. Just one of the junior doctors who came and explained, 'The test is negative, you have three options now: one, two, three. Take as much time as you need and come back to us.' I still have those papers. But I never went back. I got really attached to the people [the doctors] and then it turned out to be really commercial." What was disappointing for Amita was not only the fact that her hopes had been shattered but just as well that her doctors did not provide sufficient emotional support.

Like Amita, many patients "appeared prepared for the rigours of the discipline that the 'clinical gaze' imposed on the body, as long it was confined to the manipulation of the 'anatomical body' and did not extend to include the doctor/patient interaction. In that respect, patients sought a softening of the 'gaze'" (Bharadwaj 2016, 222). After they had spent much time in hospitals and they became familiar with their doctors, many patients felt betrayed when cycles failed. They were frustrated that doctors could not pinpoint exact reasons and provide sufficient explanations. As Dr. Nishika noted,

> I always tell them [her patients] that [positive] results are not more than
> 35 to 40 percent, and the reasons can be this, this, this. So everything has

been discussed. They already know. And yet they will ask this question. . . . But unfortunately in reproductive medicine there is nothing like this. Even when there is a clear-cut factor, like tubal factor, when the [fallopian] tubes are damaged, there can still be an implantation factor [in addition]. It is very difficult to pinpoint exactly where the problem is. You can only know that your ovarian tubes are the only problem, if your treatment is successful. . . . There are too many gray areas in reproductive medicine.

Although IVF enables the circumvention of certain problematic factors (e.g., bypassing blocked fallopian tubes), reproductive processes that are neither observable nor controllable, such as implantation, can still thwart success. Hence, it can only be verified in retrospect, after a successful treatment cycle, that the suspected factor constituted the only problem.

Since there are a lot of gray areas in reproductive medicine, as Dr. Nishika suggested, surprises occur frequently in IVF hospitals. Doctors often described the procedure as a "lottery," "gamble," or "Russian roulette" (for patients' use of gambling metaphors, see Becker 2000, 126). Sheryl de Lacey (2002, 46) points out that the metaphor of a lottery, which is also employed in IVF clinics in Australia, produces two binary subject positions: winners and losers.[12] Similarly in Delhi, with the difference that winning or losing the game was not always considered to be a mere coincidence, as Neha explained.

So many failures and on the face of it, I am not suffering from any major kind of infertility issue. Whatever I am facing is medically treatable, but still I am not able to have it. Definitely it is my destiny involved. There are people with even worse cases than me and they conceive, and I am not able to conceive. Out of ten patients probably I am one of the topmost hope-giving patients to a doctor. "She is one of the top ones, who has the highest ability of getting pregnant." But then I don't get pregnant. And I realize it is my destiny. Something is not right.

Patients as well as doctors often activate modes of retroactive ascription after IVF failures: the search for causes reaches not only back to the treatment cycle but further into the past. Failures are analyzed by referring to destiny (kismat) and karma, as connective elements between past moral responsibility and future fate that manifest in present conditions (Babb 1983, 179).[13] Dr. Bhavana, for example, stated, "We have a saying: first your destiny was written, and then your body was formed. Which means, right from the time of conception, your destiny has been written." In this sense, the infertile body constitutes a visible sign of past deeds and a site where destiny has inscribed itself.

However, this does not mean that patients stoically accept the failure of a treatment cycle as a sign of their future infertile fate. At the same time as the past has a bearing on the present, the present may influence the future. Babb (173) makes a similar point with regard to theories of misfortune that are "concerned, at least implicitly, with the future as well as the present and the past. . . . On the one hand, such a theory is retrospective, pointing backwards in time to events that shaped the present; on the other hand, it looks ahead to a future that can be influenced by actions taken now." As Dr. Bhavana explained, "Suppose you have hurt somebody in your previous life, or you've done this wrong, then you will be paying for your sins in the next life. So, there are certain things that you can do penance for. Even in this life."

Apart from reference to destiny or *karma*, god (*ūparvālā* or *bhagvān*) is also called on to explain the results of cycles. If IVF works, one patient reasoned, it is "god's way of giving you what you cannot have. We have no control. It is what it is." Another patient even deployed detailed calculations of success: "Good luck, plus strong determination, plus god's cooperation means success.

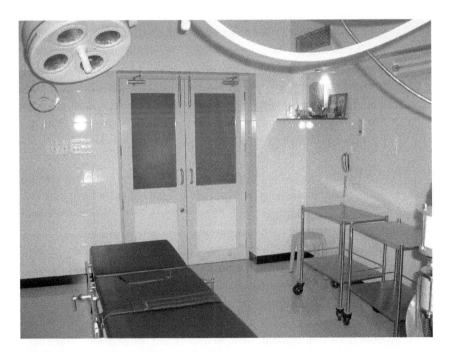

FIGURE 8. Operation theater in an IVF hospital with gods displayed in one corner. Photo by the author.

This is my equation." Doctors too invoked help during procedures and urged patients to remember god (e.g., *bhagvān ko yād karo*) for IVF to work better. Particularly the time after embryo transfer, when no further medical steps are possible and the two-week period of waiting begins, was perceived by many to be a time "where god takes over." Or, as a patient put it, "After ET [embryo transfer], everything is god or destiny."[14] In this sense, both patients and clinicians understood "the process of assisting nature itself [as in need of] assistance" (Bharadwaj 2016, 233).

And indeed, many IVF cycles fail. In these cases, doctors try to maintain the semblance of normality. They advise patients to have a break and then consult them again: "Your test is negative. Stop all medications now and wait for your period. Whenever you are ready for another cycle, come back at your second day [of the period]." However, couples often need more time to recover—not only physically but also psychologically and financially, as Amita, for example:

> This [the IVF failure] had a huge psychological impact on me. I felt frustrated. And even worse because I stay with my in-laws. They put a lot of pressure and blamed me in the sense of "you did not do this and that, maybe it would have been fine otherwise." But my husband was very supportive and patient, he also told them that they should stop. . . . My mother-in-law said immediately, "You should take another shot." And I was like, "Nobody thinks about me!" I really needed a break. It took me six to seven months to get over this. I was frustrated, went into a depression, all felt negative. I stopped praying. I put on a lot of weight and I felt really ugly and negative. Financially you can recover from this by working more, but psychologically . . .

Decisions on how to proceed take time. In the end, however, IVF often remains the only viable option for patients in their quest to establish substantial relations. This is the reason why many couples eventually return to the clinic to try once again. Amita as well started to think about another cycle, as she told me during one of our meetings: "I have now taken one and a half years of break. . . . Now I am again contemplating since the beginning of this year. Because my husband is not fine with adoption and nothing else happens. I am afraid that I will get too old and don't have the energy anymore to bring up a child." In this sense, decision-making processes often resemble cycles (Franklin 1997, 157; Wilson 2014, 2): from hope to disappointment, to doubts and deliberations, and finally to new hope and a new attempt.

Cycles of Hope

IVF trajectories usually don't end with the failure of one cycle; rather, if financial means are available, failure constitutes the starting point of a new attempt. Despite low success rates, many patients in private hospitals mobilized large amounts of money to undergo several cycles. In the public hospital, where IVF is free but pharmaceuticals are still expensive, one cycle often exhausted patients' sparse resources. And yet, people were willing to take loans or sell land and jewelry just to try one more time.

Neha

Neha was in the middle of her third IVF cycle when we had our first conversation in PremiumIVF. As she and her husband told me, they did not have a structured plan, but kept on following advice from doctors, friends, and family: "We went ahead without much thinking." Married since 2004 and trying for a child since 2005, they decided to visit a gynecologist in 2006. The initial tests indicated that Neha had a hormonal "imbalance," PCOS (polycystic ovarian syndrome, which is an endocrine disorder often associated with infertility), and one blocked tube. After nine unsuccessful cycles of ovulation induction combined with timed intercourse, Neha was referred to PremiumIVF. Like most other patients, the couple had also tried several other methods: Neha had fasted every Wednesday, she had turned vegetarian for several months, and they had gone on pilgrimages. To improve her hormonal values Neha also tried acupressure sessions for a couple of months. But in the end, she reasoned, "For us this [IVF] is the only way out."

Dr. Nishika conducted their first IVF cycle in 2007, which failed. A couple of months later Neha visited the recently opened IVF unit of CommonCare because she knew the doctor in charge. This enabled her to circumvent long lines and waiting hours. The pregnancy test, however, turned out to be negative as well. Two years later Neha and her husband decided to try IVF for a third time. They first visited a prominent doctor in Mumbai but eventually decided to conclude the cycle in PremiumIVF, which was also not successful. After this third cycle Neha decided to take a break. And, if she ever underwent IVF again, she reasoned, it would be only with donor eggs, as egg quality had been a problem in all her cycles.

Neha had a strong sense of guilt toward her husband. She regretted not being "able to give him children" and mentioned that he would have been better off if he had married another woman. While Neha's husband was more than reassuring that their childlessness would not change his feelings towards her, he still persuaded Neha to give it one more try. Thus, she underwent another IVF cycle with her own eggs in combination with LIT (lymphocyte immunization therapy) in a recently opened corporate hospital in Gurgaon, which also failed. LIT is an immunological therapy, where the white blood cells of Neha's husband are injected into her—a highly experimental and controversial therapy that is banned in several countries.

> *We had seen an ad in a newspaper offering free consultations, so my husband said we will just go and talk to them. I wasn't ready, I said no. I said, "If I want to get something done, I get a donor egg." I wasn't ready to go for a normal IVF at all. He said, "Let's go and ask, we will not go for a treatment, we will just seek opinion, what they have to say." . . . But you know, once you meet somebody and somebody gives you a shimmer of hope. Then you say, "Ok, why not." So that is the reason. And after my fourth failed attempt I said I am never going to do it again, never again. It is more than six months now and again somebody tells me why don't you try it once again. That kind of a thing. Every time I say no, but then something happens and things change.*

Although Neha had decided not to continue with fertility interventions after the fourth failure, a couple of months later doubts rose again and she contemplated another possible option: a third-party IVF cycle with donor eggs. "After four IVFs, my only hope is a donor egg. That is the only thing I have not tried yet. I just have to make up my mind to go in for a donor egg." Even though breaks between treatment cycles had grown larger, the thought about trying continued to emerge. "Most likely, if I have to again think about it, I will go in for donor, not my own eggs anymore. . . . This is what is on my mind, this is on the agenda for this year. I am going to turn thirty-six now, so it is time to make decisions."

What prompts patients like Neha to spend an enormous amount of time and resources on a procedure as uncertain as IVF? Neha cited the "shimmer of hope" that compelled her to undergo cycle after cycle. "If I have hope," she told me, "I would do it. If I even have 10 percent hope, I would do it." Hope is palpable in various ways when visiting IVF hospitals, for example in the form of (sometimes exaggerated) success rates that manage to translate an uncertain event into a tangible figure. Hope is further nourished by thank-you cards from patients and photographs of babies, all neatly pinned to the walls of waiting rooms. Slogans, such as "Yes! You can have a baby" or "Way to parenthood made easy" are also frequently displayed in clinics.

Although "[t]o have or to 'live in' hope means to take an active stance towards the future so that the possibilities and potentiality inherent in the present may be rendered achievable" (Novas 2006, 291), hope constitutes a double-edged sword

for IVF patients: "enabling women to continue and dis-abling them from reach-
ing an endpoint of treatment" (Franklin 1997, 192). I have to note, however, that
doctors in PremiumIVF and CommonCare did not explicitly "sell hope" (Becker
2000, 116) in consultations but made an effort to downplay patients' expectations. "It is not like using a credit card: you don't dip the card and immediately
get a baby," Dr. Isha explained. I often witnessed fierce discussions when she
tried to make clear to patients that there is no guarantee for a positive outcome:
"It is so difficult to make them understand that this is not 100 percent," fumed
Dr. Isha after such a consultation. And Dr. Nishika continuously emphasized that
IVF cannot be called an efficient treatment, almost so that she as a clinician has
lost hope in it:

> I think the [medical] understanding even in so many years has not pro-
> gressed as it should, and we are still very much behind in calling it [IVF]
> an efficient treatment. It is not an efficient treatment. Any treatment
> which doesn't even give 50 percent results, you can hardly call it effi-
> cient. So there is a lot more to understand before we can say, "Yes, this is
> it, you know. This is it, what we are offering will give the patient a good
> hope of pregnancy." So we are not there yet. . . . It started with a lot of
> hope, but then over the years we haven't moved fast.

But physicians also justified practicing IVF, despite its uncertainty, through the
few successful cases they were able to enter in the books. Dr. Aishwa, for example, explained that "inability to conceive is something very stressful and very
demoralizing for the patient. And unfortunately, success is not 100 percent. But
at least we have to try. At least we made a few [patients] pregnant, which otherwise would not have become pregnant."

Whether doctors explicitly sell hope or not, it is fueled at any rate through the
temporal logic of successive cycles. Treatment cycles don't unfold in a repetitive
way. Rather, clinicians make sure to always change a feature or add another technique during a new cycle in order to demonstrate progress, such as LIT in Neha's
case. And the possibilities of add-ons are numerous: different ovarian stimulation protocols, ICSI, donor gametes, or surrogacy arrangements. "There are so
many options now of trying for a child, which always provide a ray of hope. If
this does not work, then there is donation or surrogacy and all different combina-
tions," explained Neha. New techniques incite new hope that it might work this
time with this particular procedure. This mixture of promise and hope prompts
many patients to embark on one IVF cycle after another. And since hope hardly
ever loosens its grip, it leaves them stuck in a vortex of treatment cycles, failures,
and new trials.

Time to Stop

Similar to infertility as an experience "out of synchrony" (Becker 2000, 117) or as a liminal period from which couples cannot move on to parenthood, IVF itself creates another form of liminality (Franklin 1997): many patients get caught in a series of treatment cycles from which they can only extricate themselves through their own decision to stop. Most clinicians do *not* explicitly tell patients to end interventions, as Dr. Lakshmi exemplified. "I always tell the patient, 'You have come to me with a desire, not with a disease. And it is up to you to what extent you want to go ahead and fulfill your desire. *You* have to draw the line.'" For patients, however, this proves to be a tricky endeavor. "The paradox at the heart of this quest for conception is that, while the infertile critique medical interventions as unsatisfactory, they continue to endure them in the absence of any tangible alternatives" (Bharadwaj 2016, 211).

When I contacted patients one or two years after I had first met them in IVF clinics, I was surprised at first that most of those who were still childless were willing to talk to me again. During our conversations I realized that they did so because IVF was not a closed chapter in their lives. They deliberated whether to go for another IVF cycle, add another feature, or try another doctor. They pondered over possible reasons why it had not worked for them, and they were curious about my opinion regarding hospitals. Even when people had decided to go ahead with adoption, short interjections like, "maybe we should have tried once again," made it clear that the idea of IVF had not been shelved completely. Sometimes, this led to apparently retrograde decisions. Couples who had already set their mind on adoption or who had already adopted a child returned to IVF clinics only to try once more, hoping to finally succeed in their quest for substantial relations. The few people I met who were able to stop IVF were the ones who either eventually had a child or suffered severe complications from the procedure.

Urshita

Urshita was one of the few patients whose IVF cycles had failed but who had made peace with her reproductive trajectory. She was able to do so because she eventually conceived on her own and had a son. She was one of those so-called miracle cases where conception happened naturally after failed IVF cycles.[15]

This was the third time Urshita had invited me to her house—a different one each time. It seemed that she keeps on moving with her husband and her father-in-law from one housing society to the other within the newly developing areas of the National Capital Region. The construction of the apartment block in which they were living at that time was not yet finished. Gray walls awaited their whitewash, and the shopping and sport facilities were still far from being inaugurated. Their decision to buy this apartment had happened all of a sudden, Urshita told me, "like everything in my life." Another instance where Urshita's resoluteness had manifested itself was when her family arranged for her marriage in a middle-sized town at the foothills of the Himalayas. The agent they had employed was supposed to propose several suitable candidates to her and her family. Urshita, however, liked the first man whose profile she saw and decided to stop her search right there.

Similarly, Urshita maintained her firm decision not to undertake any more attempts after one fresh and one frozen failed IVF cycle. The day she learned that her second pregnancy test (from the frozen embryo transfer) was negative, she was so disappointed that she remained in the car while her husband and mother sat through the session with the doctors, who recommended that she undertake another attempt one month later. When she called me after a few days to tell me about the result, she had already made up her mind not to follow this advice. "I need a break. I have taken medications for two years now. There are side effects. Doctors take the easy way and tell you to try it again. But they don't have to take the injections. It is burdensome, also emotionally and psychologically. And it is expensive." Taking this decision was by no means an easy task. Urshita's mother-in-law, who had been living with them, had often articulated her wish to see the child of her only son. And maybe Urshita would have thought about another attempt if she had not conceived naturally after a few months—despite her diagnosis of blocked tubes.

Seven years after her wedding, she gave birth to a son. Her husband was still agitated over the fact that the doctors had told them that they could not conceive naturally. He was tempted to return to the hospital to show their son as a vivid proof of their error. Urshita, however, tried to forget those difficult times filled with hospital visits and medications. "I don't want to think about IVF anymore. Those were dark times." It was noticeable though that Urshita refused to be determined by her past IVF experience in decisions about her future reproductive trajectory. Shortly after the birth of her son, Urshita got pregnant again, much to her surprise. She and her husband were not sure whether they wanted another child. Further, the "spacing" to their first son seemed too narrow to them. Spacing—the temporal distance between children—is an important aspect in family planning in India. Therefore, they decided to abort and try for another child later. "If it happens, fine, if not then we have him," Urshita concluded.

There are, however, IVF failures that do not end as happily as Urshita's story. Tara, for example, was one of the few women who completely broke with IVF without conceiving, because of severe side effects. Often neglected is the fact that IVF includes not only the risk of failure but also the risk of major health complications.[16]

Tara

Tara met her husband, Kapil, during their college days. They married a few years later, but were not particularly keen on having children right away even though there was a lot of pressure from Kapil's parents, as their only other son and his wife had problems conceiving. However, as soon as they found out about Tara's PCOS during a routine check-up, they started consulting doctors: "Initially for me, because also there was an issue [with infertility] for Kapil's brother, there was kind of a pressure on me. From day one of my marriage I was told that 'you get us a baby, make us grandparents.' We did not take it very seriously. But after we found out about PCOS we actually pressed the panic button. So yes, I wanted to conceive and I wanted to become a mother. That was the logical next step for us."

After several stimulated and monitored cycles as well as a couple of IUIs that remained unsuccessful, Tara had been preparing very diligently for her IVF cycle in a private clinic in Gurgaon, a satellite city of Delhi and part of the National Capital Region: she had stopped smoking, taken leave from her job, and aligned her daily schedule to injection timings. When I met her for the first time through a common friend, she was extremely optimistic and looked forward to this new option that would help her become pregnant. However, during the treatment cycle, Tara had to be admitted to the hospital with OHSS (ovarian hyperstimulation syndrome). OHSS is one of the possible risks recorded on informed consent forms and recited quickly to every patient before the procedure. Resulting from high doses of hormonal pharmaceuticals, it can become life-threatening.

Almost two years later, Tara recalled the events that led to her failed IVF cycle: everything seemed to be perfectly fine until the embryo transfer. Her doctor was content with the number of egg cells and praised the morphology of the embryos as looking "just as in science books." But the morning after her embryo transfer Tara started to complain about breathlessness to her husband, who immediately took her to the hospital. Tara remembered, "They said it is alright, it happens at times, take a puff or two. Then I came back home. Two days later again I had a very major attack, and I was rushed back and admitted. Dr. Vibhuti is the gynecologist, and her husband is a physician [who treated her for OHSS]. I still remember that I was concerned about the baby, in case there is any development, but he said, 'No, my first priority now is to save your life.' Because there was a lot of water. They took out seven liters of water from my body, from my lungs and other cavities." After a few days, Tara recovered. Her pregnancy test, however, turned out to be negative.

Furthermore, all the costs resulting from the complications had to be borne by Tara and Kapil—a considerable expense. Tara's disappointment was still visible in the way she stored her medical reports in her apartment in Gurgaon. While all her pre-IVF records were neatly arranged, and she had even drawn up a table with dates of interventions and prescribed medications, the papers of her IVF cycle were cluttered and had started going moldy. "This was for the IVF. I never touched this bag again," she remarked while trying to sort through the papers.

IVF not only constituted a medical disappointment but had greater repercussions on Tara's life: for a few months after the treatment Tara suffered from severe acne, and she also gained a lot of weight. She was contemplating quitting her job when her boss started delaying her salary, but she stayed on because she knew that a new employer might not grant her the necessary leaves, if she ever wanted to go for another IVF cycle. When I met her, Tara seemed hopeless and directionless: "I feel like my life is at standstill at the moment. Usually you have something to look forward to: college, careers, children. But I have the feeling that there is nothing for me right now." She reaffirmed this feeling a year later when she reflected about this time: "There was nothing to look forward to, and that is a sad feeling. I used to at times feel that my life is just this, it should end now. Not that I was getting suicidal, but I felt that whatever I had to do in my life is done, now it is one drag."

Even though Tara is still not sure about how to proceed, she is certain that she will never try IVF again. "You saw me in a bad phase of my life," she told me several years after the incident. "I will not do this to myself and my body anymore. Then I was in a huge mental agony. I am still trying to come out of it, mentally and physically. It took also a toll on Kapil and me as a couple. It is a huge cost that I paid."

Although Tara managed to stop IVF, it proved to be a painful process. Since it implies the opportunity for a new beginning, failure paradoxically constitutes "the force through which dreams and desires for the future are renewed" (Cross 2014, 23). Hence, rejecting a new attempt at IVF, even after failed cycles, is tantamount to shattering one's dreams and contenting oneself with an alternative future, devoid of substantial relations.

Although clearly exaggerated, the "IVF success rates," as they were displayed in a private hospital in Delhi, guide patients in their quest for substantial relations. Generating hope, the logic of success rates seduces patients to proceed with medical interventions. But the establishment of genealogical continuity through IVF is rarely straightforward. As the five narratives have shown, reproductive trajectories of infertile couples cannot be understood as progressive flows toward a fertile future; rather, they constitute convoluted and onerous paths that are infused with negative temporalities.

In addition to describing patients' relationship to IVF over time, the chapter observed how IVF cycles unfold in specific rhythms. I demonstrated how clinical interventions, such as ovarian stimulation, are designed to manipulate female bodies in order to make them productive and valuable for IVF. However, bodies do not simply obey medical practice but respond and interfere—they "kick back" (Barad 1998, 112). Or, as Emilia Sanabria (2016) put it, bodies are plastic: malleable *and* resisting. They make their presence felt in clinical life through different modes of somatic activity that materialize in the form of temporality, productivity, and unpredictability.[17] Bodies' engagement with medical practice during ovarian stimulation demands responsiveness from physicians and may compel them to attune to somatic rhythms—a topic to which I return in chapter 6. In the next chapter, I argue that IVF is not only valued but also feared for its promise to generate substantial relations.

WHEN CELLS CIRCULATE
Unwanted Ties

"My wife and I are looking for a suitable sperm donor for fresh In Vitro procedure very soon! Ideal candidate should be IIT student [Indian Institute of Technology, an elite educational institution], healthy, no bad habits, tall and fair if possible but will consider the right donor regardless of looks etc." This advertisement appeared in an Indian online forum in 2012. The couple's idea of a candidate articulates bluntly what many patients in IVF clinics or donor agencies request more furtively: "suitable" donors. It hints at the fact that third-party reproduction in India is a delicate affair that is characterized by concerns about using substances from "outside" a specific group. Particularly the establishment of substantial relations that run contrary to endogamous norms is regarded with skepticism in IVF centers in Delhi.

The circulation of reproductive substances in IVF hospitals is further linked to moral panics about inappropriate forms of mixing on a larger scale, as is reflected in an online comment posted as a response to an article of an Indian news outlet discussing gamete donations: "What if the marriage between kids of donated [donors] and received [recipients] happens? Will it not [be] tantamount to incest? . . . This can potentially become a time bomb where you end up [with a] specific set of donors, controlled by sperm bank which can carefully plant sperm of a specific caste/religion (kind of high-tech conversion) . . . This is a dangerous trend. This can create lots of property dispute and may create more chaos." The commentator paints a dystopian vision of dispute and chaos through the movement of gametes outside familial bonds, leading to—in their

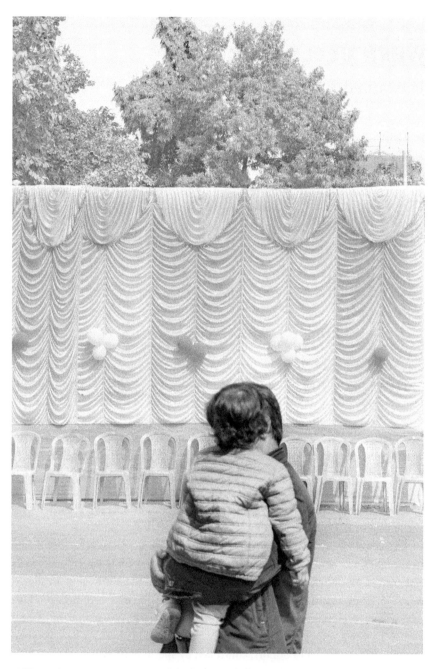

FIGURE 9. Father and child at an IVF event. Photo by Chhandak Pradhan.

view—inappropriate relations on a societal level: incestuous marriages, transgressions of caste boundaries, or even "high-tech conversion."

As we have seen, IVF has the power to establish substantial relations. In an ideal form, it produces offspring within conjugal relationships and continues a patrilineage. But reproductive technologies have also made possible novel forms of reproduction, for example through third-party IVF cycles (i.e., the use of donor gametes). While, in some parts of the world, IVF is celebrated for this ability to establish nonnormative connections, it often constitutes a cause for concern in India. In this chapter, I explore what happens when cells circulate in IVF clinics in Delhi, with a particular focus on anxieties about unwanted ties. In a first step, I show how middle-class patients who are medically advised to use donor gametes are wary about substances from spheres outside their familial circles. They fear mismatches leading to the transgression of boundaries that are not to be transgressed in a highly stratified society. Gamete recipients therefore conceal possible normative breaches through attempts to establish continuity and secrecy. Second, IVF patients more generally are concerned about accidental mix-ups in IVF centers. Many interlocutors worried about the fact that gametes travel from the body to the laboratory and back, a trajectory that makes them susceptible to mistakes. Depicting rumors and practices of gamete sharing in low-cost hospitals, I demonstrate that particularly working-class patients are subjected to regimes of gamete circulations they can hardly control. Finally, I argue that anxieties connected to IVF point to wider moral panics about socio-moral deterioration in contemporary urban India.

Substantial Transactions

In order to understand fears about gamete mixing in IVF hospitals, I return to discussions about the relational potential of substances. The exchange of substances has constituted a long-standing concern in the anthropological literature on kinship and relatedness in South Asia. Pioneered by McKim Marriott, scholars of the Chicago school of ethnosociology have illustrated how daily interactions are consequential in that they create and maintain forms of relatedness through the exchange of substances. Central in Marriott's description of "transactional thinking in South Asian, Hindu society" is the notion of "substance-code": "natural matter, actions, words and thoughts are all substances and all imbued with relational properties" (Marriott 1990, 2).[1] It is exactly because substances are imbued with relational properties that their unconventional circulation elicits anxieties. Substances are understood to transmit formative qualities, as they have the power to "reproduce in others something of the nature of the persons in whom they have originated" (Marriott 1976, 111). While in daily life sharing food and engaging in sexual relationships are the most intimate and potentially dangerous forms of interaction, IVF offers novel but similarly threatening types of substantial exchanges: Gametes are endowed with the power to connect not only parents and children but also donors and recipients (for "relations of non-relations" in the United Kingdom, see Konrad 2005).

Another important facet of Marriott's work is his analysis of substantial transactions as closely linked to status and social stratification in North India: transactions not only express but also produce hierarchical differentiations. Caste hierarchies, for example, regulate exchanges, and they, in turn, are based on the exchange of substance-codes. Because inappropriate forms of interaction may result in adulteration and impurity, there are different transactional strategies for different caste groups according to Marriott's ideal-typical scheme. By and large, higher castes can interact in a controlled manner, while the status of lower castes is characterized by uncontrollability. Helen Lambert (2000), however, shows how such rules may be subverted in order to create nonnormative forms of relatedness. In Rajasthan, daily practices of affection and nurturance establish "optative" relations running counter to conventional lines of kinship or caste distinctions. As transactions of substance-codes imply the simultaneous transformation of the exchange parties involved, they may constitute a deliberate strategy in processes of doing relatedness. Lambert's compelling account is part of a larger strand of scholarship—often termed new kinship studies—which diverges from understandings of kinship as "an aftereffect of the natural facts of sexual reproduction" (Franklin and McKinnon 2001, 2).[2]

Although a welcome antithesis to the almost exclusive occupation with descent or alliance during a large part of the discipline's history, the view of relatedness as negotiated, flexible, or optative carries the danger of neglecting normativity (Miller 2007). Not "any relationship can also be made postnatally or performatively by culturally appropriate action," Marshall Sahlins (2013, 2) warns. Moreover, in his insightful analysis of reproductive technologies, Morgan Clarke (2008, 158) adds that new kinship studies, "where they express an interest in the questioning of received moral categories, can be seen as intimately bound up in a historical movement of liberal reform of the institutions of personal status, relations between the sexes, and sexual morality." In many contexts, third-party IVF cycles have been interpreted as an opportunity to transcend limiting boundaries and create new possibilities of relatedness. But "while assisted reproduction has brought some people increased freedom and opportunity . . . advances in reproductive technology too have promoted and maintained certain power relations, notions of gender, and particular constructions of the family"

(Deomampo 2016, 6; see also Franklin 2013). For example, Clarke explains how gamete donations in Lebanon mainly carry connotations of immorality. For this reason, relations are hidden if they are conceived to be outside registers of "sexual propriety." In India too, the inclusion of third parties is not necessarily regarded as liberating or desirable. A technology with the capacity to transgress boundaries and undermine hierarchies rather elicits moral panics in a highly stratified society. In the following sections, I discuss two forms of mixing that are regarded with skepticism because of their capacity to establish nonnormative substantial relations: mismatches during third-party IVF cycles and uncontrolled laboratory mix-ups in IVF hospitals.

Mismatches

Mixing reproductive substances beyond familial boundaries may be a deliberate process, for example when patients are recommended to undergo an IVF cycle using sperm or egg cells from gamete donors. For most patients, however, this proves to be problematic medical advice, since it implies that reproductive substances from third parties enter an intimate process. As Bharadwaj (2003, 1868) notes, the inclusion of a third party "fractures culturally conceptualized boundaries of a family as inextricably tied to the conjugal bond." Moreover, donor gametes might establish substantial relations that are interpreted as unconventional and inappropriate.

Donor Substances

While third-party cycles in general evoke discomfort among most patients using IVF facilities, concerns differ depending on the biological substances involved.[3] Sperm donation is often described as particularly unsettling, for two reasons. Firstly, constituting a "cross-sex" relationship (Bergmann 2014, 131), sperm donation may give rise to accusations of adultery or prostitution. This is exacerbated by the fact that most female patients visiting private hospitals supposedly are of a higher social status than sperm donors, thereby reversing common practices of hypergamy. Secondly, semen is regarded as *the* important vehicle for descent. "Sperm is important," one patient remarked. "Otherwise it is a different child." Many others concurred that if sperm was derived from someone else, the resulting child would not be one's "own," because semen transmits the "blood" of the lineage. This reflects a patrilineal understanding of kinship in which— as another patient explained—"the descent line [vanś] goes through the male.

The family name should continue, and this is possible only through one's own sperm." For this reason patients in need of donor sperm occasionally requested their doctors to use semen from the brother-in-law or father-in-law of the female patient. Whereas some doctors outrightly rejected this request on the grounds of bioethical guidelines (see also Bharadwaj 2016, 151), others were sympathetic to it because it mirrors practices of levirate marriage (for Sri Lanka, see Simpson 2004a, 164; for Lebanon, see M. Clarke 2009, 169) and resembles popular adoption practices in which children are passed on within the extended family. As Dr. Lakshmi argued, "The social framework is very different for different families. We have cases here in Haryana [a neighboring state of Delhi] where once a woman loses her husband, when she is widowed, she is not sent out of the family. She marries her brother-in-law. If there is no brother-in-law, she marries her father-in-law. That is the society, that is the norm."

While, at first, many patients reject donor sperm from outside familiar circles, egg donation is considered to be less problematic, since—as one patient put it—"in eggs, nothing comes, like characteristics, genes."[4] This is hardly surprising considering predominant understandings of reproduction in North India: "In patrilineal India the commonly-held idea regarding the roles of father and mother in procreation is that the man provides the seed—the essence—while the woman provides the field which receives the seed and nourishes it" (Dube 1988, WS11). Reproduction thus constitutes a process to which both partners contribute unequally, as it is "the seed that determines social identity. The seed is the source of life, the field in turn merely nurtures that life" (Patel 2007, 33). Yet, despite the indisputable importance of the "seed," many women I met emphasized their own substantial contributions to the reproductive process through carrying, nourishing, and giving birth to the child. They were ready to accept egg cells from donors because they deemed their own contributions through substantial transactions during pregnancy much more relevant. "It [egg donation] doesn't make a difference. The blood is my own. What is important is that I give birth to it," said one woman. Providing nourishing blood for the fetus in her womb during pregnancy would turn a child conceived through egg donation into her own, another patient explained: "It doesn't matter, it stays in my womb [god] for nine months, blood [khūn] and bones [haḍḍī] will be made from my food and drink" (see also Bennett 1983; Böck and Rao 2000; Pande 2009; Vora 2013; Bärnreuther 2018). In contrast to biogenetic understandings, it is not only gametes that matter. Formative substances, such as blood or later milk, also contribute to the development of the child and, consequently, the establishment of maternity. Although most patients clearly accept donor egg cells more easily than donor sperm, reservations against all kinds of mixing are common.

Flexible Norms

When patients receive medical advice to use donor gametes, most worry about the generation of substantial relations deviating from normative frameworks. Many therefore do not consent to donor cycles at first but undergo several trials of IVF with their own gametes. Patients' accounts about their decisions to *not* use donor gametes were often mediated by religious and moral concerns regarding the "unnaturalness" of the procedure, sexual propriety, and understandings of descent and heredity. Many Muslim patients assured me that they would undergo IVF only using their own gametes. Shabnam, for example, explained, "It is forbidden to take [gametes] from outside." This coincides with Marcia Inhorn's (2006, 427) observation in Egypt, where, "as early as 1980, authoritative fatwas issued from [the] famed Al-Azhar University suggested that IVF and similar technologies are permissible as long as they do not involve any form of third-party donation" (for the unproblematic use of donor gametes in Iran, a Shia-dominated country, see Abbasi-Shavazi et al. 2008). Many Christian patients were similarly skeptical about IVF in general and third-party options in particular. Moreover, despite the fact that Hindu patients never referred to any specific religious restrictions, most would nevertheless first try to conceive with their own gametes. However, the fact that I met Muslims, Christians, and Hindus who eventually used third-party donations after failed IVF cycles with their own gametes suggests that norms are flexible.

Understandings of what kinds of procedures are permissible and what kinds of transgressions justifiable change over patients' treatment trajectories (Becker 2000, 68). Sheryl, a Catholic, was aware of the church's opposition to assisted reproductive technologies (see, for example, Ratzinger and Bovone 1987). Yet, she used IVF and even consented to a donor cycle after she had remained childless for fourteen years. "It is a hard reality, and you have to make your choice. I am a very religious person, but I made my own choice. And I don't see anything wrong. It's not that I do prostitution. It's more like blood donation: you don't have something and you get it." Justifying her choice to use donor eggs, Sheryl compared egg donation to blood donation in order to prevent possible interpretations of her third-party cycle as sexually improper (prostitution). Similarly, many patients eventually agree to undergo an IVF cycle in combination with third-party substances after cycles with their own gametes have kept on failing.[5]

Silent Breaches

Once they take this decision, patients have two options: to use known donors, usually from within their own family, or to use unknown, commercial donors.[6]

Since many couples are concerned about the transgression of social boundaries, they prefer gametes from intrafamilial donors, for example, using sperm of a male agnatic kin or egg cells from a female uterine kin. Anindita Majumdar (2017, 93) adds that acceptable candidates for egg donation or surrogacy are also those women who fit "the Indo-Aryan kinship practice of the flow of women in one direction." However, the latest Assisted Reproductive Technology (Regulation) Bill stipulates that "clinics shall obtain donor gametes from [ART] banks" (Government of India 2020, 8), which effectively rules out donations from known donors. This will make third-party IVF cycles unaffordable and/or unacceptable for many patients. Various clinicians and policy makers, however, argued that this provision prevents possible coercion to donate within families as well as emotional challenges or property disputes that might arise later on. For exactly this reason, some patients mentioned that they avoided requesting gametes from family members. They feared fights in case regrets or envy were to plague their donors later. In other cases, they explained that gamete donation would constitute a debt too high to repay. They tried to avoid constant feelings of guilt toward someone close to them by searching for distant and commercial donors.

The second option is so-called commercial donors, who receive a payment for their services—an option that is viable only for middle-class patients in the case of egg cells (as they are quite expensive). When interlocutors referred to gametes from unknown, commercial donors, they employed the expressions "from someone else" (*kisī aur se*) or "from outside" (*bāhar se*). "From outside" denotes spheres beyond one's own family but also beyond caste or religious boundaries. And indeed, the transgression of endogamous norms is highly likely during commercial third-party IVF cycles. With the exception of few "premium donor" programs or "diva donors" (Deomampo 2016, 107), most gamete donors are from low socioeconomic backgrounds and not compatible with the high expectations of those middle-class patients who are able to afford this rather expensive procedure. Recipients thus have to come to terms with the fact that the "quality" of donors (Wahlberg 2008; Mohr 2018) does not meet their requirements (for strategies of hospitals to mediate these concerns and maintain an illusion of suitability, see Bärnreuther 2018; for the concealment of organ donor biographies, see also Sharp 2001).

For this reason, most patients who eventually decided to use gametes from commercial donors did not disclose this fact to family and friends, in the hope that their commitment to secrecy would help to socially emplace their future child in kinship networks (Bharadwaj 2016; for the "social process of fabricating nonrelatedness," see Kahn 2000, 165). "Otherwise people might not accept it as our child," was the widespread reasoning. Although children conceived through donor gametes are recognized legally, gamete recipients argued that only silence would help to turn their child into a legitimate offspring and heir. This is reminiscent of Veena Das's description of abducted women who returned to their families after the subcontinent's partition. They could be reabsorbed into family structures "as long as the breaches of norms could be covered by veils of silence" (1995, 218). In a similar way, nonnormative connections introduced via IVF are obscured through secrecy and a "narrative of conventionality" (M. Clarke 2008, 164)—that is, natural conception or IVF with a couple's own gametes.[7] The moral imperative to silence (for the moral imperative to transparency in the United Kingdom, see Strathern 1999) has been facilitated by the *National Guidelines*, which assure anonymity between commercial donors and recipients. Yet the attempt to completely erase these relations can never be successful. "[L]ike the repressed, biology returns" (Laqueur 2000, 92). Specters may haunt recipients later on, for instance through the possibility of incestuous relations (see below).[8]

Curating Connections

In addition to silencing nonnormative relations, recipients try to carefully curate connections when they use commercial gamete donors, starting with the search for "suitable substances" (Bärnreuther 2018; for curating race, see also Moll 2019). Doctors or agents provide couples with biodata sheets of possible donors that contain information about physical and social characteristics and sometimes even photographs. In the process of choosing, most couples are concerned about their donor's physical appearance, usually foregrounding skin color (Whittaker and Speier 2010, 378; for racial reproductive imaginaries in transnational surrogacy arrangements, see also Deomampo 2016). With skin color being defined "along a spectrum of shades" (Deomampo 2016, 100), from "dark" to "wheatish" to "fair," donor gametes are "valued in an economy of color reflective of a history of colonialism and racism" (110). Doctors sometimes joked about the—in their view too "ambitious"—wishes of patients who requested donors with fair skin color. One embryologist even reported about patients' complaints that reach him now and then, when a baby conceived by donor gametes appeared too dark to the parents after birth. But a donor deemed suitable is not necessarily the most light-skinned donor. Striving for "corporeal continuity" (Klotz 2014), parents search for resemblance (Burghardt and Tote 2010; Mamo 2005)—a reason why they usually choose the lightest skin color still similar to their own. As one woman stated, "Looks and color are important, not like black and also not very fair. Like me." Resemblance ensures the invisibility of inappropriate substantial relations and the acceptance of the child as one's "own."

Along with physical continuity, recipients are also in search of social continuity. The "promise of inheritable phenotypic and skin color characteristics"
(Deomampo 2016, 101) is supplemented by further characteristics deemed relevant for hereditary transmission, such as caste, education, or religion. "It should
be the same kind as we, same caste, good education," explained one patient. "Family background" or "moral and cultural values" (*sanskār*) often served as euphe-
misms for requesting a donor of one's own caste. Of course, opinions differed,
and other patients forcefully rejected the idea of matching caste, especially those
who themselves had unconventional life partners: "Caste is not important, my
marriage is also intercaste." Even more than caste, many patients mentioned that
they prefer donors of their own religion. Others, however, objected and explained
that "education would be the first thing [that is important in a donor], because
it is in our hands after god decides in which direction he sets us. Religion is not
in our hands."

Requests regarding suitable substances reveal the manifold assumptions of
what kinds of characteristics are transmittable and therefore relevant—not only
among patients but also among clinicians and agents. One egg donor agent, for
example, usually tried to match religion and caste between donors and recipients.
If she could not provide a donor of the corresponding *jāti*, she at least tried to
couple vegetarian donors with vegetarian recipients. "Even though it is not in the
cells whether you are a vegetarian, people still think it matters. They think it is
transmitted by the blood," she explained. The director of a sperm bank, on the
other hand, maintained that gametes do not have any caste or religion: "We are
talking science. It is not in my blood. I could have been a Muslim had my parents
been Muslims. It is your influence that is important. This is the same in adoption.
The values you teach are important." Thus, questions of hereditary transmission
are posed and answered in a variety of ways. And these answers matter, as they
either ascertain continuity for patients or highlight a rupture.

Engineered Socialities

While many, particularly middle-class, interlocutors foregrounded the threats
entailed in processes of mixing, a few doctors regarded it as an opportunity.
Scaling up from an individual or familial level and envisioning broader societal
consequences, they considered specific forms of mixing as a powerful tool to
substantially engineer ideal socialities. I introduce two doctors who imagined
being able to improve the nation and its population by mixing reproductive
substances—either along or across social fault lines.

Dr. Manish, an embryologist in a pricey corporate hospital, viewed controlled
gamete mixings as a possibility to "better society." Rather than relying only on

semen provided by commercial sperm banks (which he perceived to be of low quality), he persuaded some of the male doctors of his hospital to become sperm donors. Dr. Manish perceived his efforts to recruit "elite" donors as a way to propagate "better" biological material and, ultimately, contribute to national improvement. "We don't do cobbler, washermen [occupations connected to a low caste status], . . . so you can better the society," he reasoned.[9] Moreover, he reserved these samples for well-off, or in his words "exclusive," patients. "Some people are a class above the rest. And you come to know they will not accept any average sample. And it is justified also. They can afford, they can pay, so why not, why not a better sample?" Employing elaborate strategies to ensure what he considered to be appropriate transactions, Dr. Manish strongly supported stratified forms of mixing.

While Dr. Manish tried to "better society" by holding on to normative frameworks, Dr. Rohit relished the idea of transgressing boundaries through the circulation of reproductive substances. An embryologist in another corporate hospital, Dr. Rohit regarded the anxieties of his middle-class patients as a missed opportunity to build integrative socialities (for another kind of "utopian somatics," see Alter 1992; or for a "political aesthetic of integration," see Copeman and Banerjee 2019). He attributed his clients' sense of ownership over their gametes to a possessive mentality. "Earlier, there were multiple marriages. Now it is only *my* family, in the sense of me and my husband. Earlier, there was also adoption in the sense that one donated to relatives. Now this is not allowed." He was pleased about the state's lethargy toward introducing the Assisted Reproductive Technology (Regulation) Bill, which would monitor hospitals more strictly, and interpreted it with the then government's commitment to the theme "Unity in Diversity." "They don't really mind gamete sharing, in fact they support genetic mismatching," he suggested, implying that a copious circulation of gametes would be endorsed by the state by way of nonregulation. Dr. Rohit imagined the government promoting mix-ups as a way to advance unity, thereby "espousing the older Nehruvian inclusive and integrative idea of a national sociality" (D. Banerjee 2011, 490; see also Copeman 2013, 202)—almost a biomedical way of nation-building whereby caste and class divisions are obliterated. Although Dr. Rohit could not act on his vision at his workplace in a corporate hospital, his ideas were sometimes echoed in rationalizations of egg sharing in low-cost clinics.

Although mismatches are inevitable as donors and recipients are usually of different social status, commercial third-party IVF cycles in pricey corporate hospitals constitute a relatively *controlled* form of mixing for middle-class patients (or, at least, they provide an illusion of control; Bärnreuther 2018). By curating and silencing relations, seemingly inappropriate ties and the concomitant breach of social norms can be avoided or hidden (J. Edwards 2014). However, there are also forms of *uncontrolled* circulations in IVF hospitals, to which mainly working-class patients are subjected.

Out of Control

Anxieties and suspicions about uncontrolled forms of mixing in IVF clinics in Delhi appear in manifold guises. I first describe the fear of *accidental* gamete mix-ups that many IVF patients harbor. Later, I turn to rumors and practices of *intentional* redistribution of egg cells in low-cost hospitals.

Accidental Mix-Ups

"After I came back from the [embryo] transfer today, the first thing my mother asked me was, 'Did you check whether they put [in] *your* eggs [embryos]?'" a patient I had met in PremiumIVF told me after her embryo transfer. Her mother's question reveals the concerns about uncontrolled, accidental mix-ups in IVF laboratories that many patients harbor. And they are not completely unfounded: several accidental mix-ups have indeed happened in various countries (e.g., Spriggs 2003) and were also widely reported in Indian media. While a few patients insisted on inspecting the laboratory setup or on the spouse being present during embryo transfer to feel assured that no mix-ups would happen (see also Kahn 2000; Inhorn 2003b), most chose to trust their doctors. "If you do something out of the ordinary [IVF]," one patient argued, "then you should trust the person. Not monitor and think whether embryos are mine or not. We trust the doctor like a god, it is one of the noblest profession. And as you cannot question your god, you cannot question your doctor. They will do the best from their side. And they also take an oath, what is it called? Like the army people to serve the people of their country without taking any personal interests. So there are values. The rest is fortune."

The addendum "the rest is fortune" nevertheless points to a certain sense of unease about IVF. Not everyone does indeed trust their doctors (see below), and many patients wonder what happens when gametes move through the laboratory, a space outside their control. Clinicians counteract these apprehensions by naturalizing IVF (see also Franklin 1997). They assure patients that fertilization in the lab happens "just like inside the body," thereby rhetorically extending the realm of the familiar inside to the threatening outside. Along these lines, embryologists emphasize their efforts to maintain laboratory conditions that resemble the in vivo environment of the body as closely as possible (see chapter 6). Further, they affirm their compliance with laboratory protocols designed to contain biologicals within demarcated spaces and prevent mix-ups (for containment in laboratories, see Mohr 2016). For example, as soon as reproductive substances enter the laboratory, embryologists attach labels to the containers in which they are located and the equipment with which they are handled. Biologicals of different patients are stored in different corners of the incubator, and their trajectories, which might include a stop at the cryopreservation unit, are meticulously registered in laboratory records.

Although I never asked directly about the implementation of good laboratory practice in my discussions with clinicians and embryologists, many interlocutors offered statements akin to this: "In our hospital, there is no foul play, patients only receive their own gametes. Everything is very open." Such comments were usually followed by a reference to the hospital's commitment to the *National Guidelines* and the Assisted Reproductive Technology (Regulation) Bill (see also Deomampo 2016, 106). Moreover, physicians' reassurances about their clinics' own good medical practice were sometimes accompanied by rumors about practices of uncontrolled mixing in other hospitals. No matter whether true or not, these rumors prove to be valuable ethnographic sources because they are shaped by "norms of what should or could be, and . . . by social constructions of danger and threat" (Eckert 2012, 154).

Rumors of Redistribution

When I first met Dr. Dipti, she promised to tell me "everything" about IVF in India. After Dr. Dipti had been educated as a gynecologist in India, she received additional training in embryology at a university hospital in Europe but eventually decided to return to India. She mentioned that after several years of practice abroad, she had to adjust to how things were done in India. On a foggy winter evening—the conference season had just begun—Dr. Dipti offered me a ride home after an IVF conference in South Delhi. Grateful for the opportunity to finally talk to one of the busiest embryologists in town, I immediately inquired about the differences between practices in Indian and foreign embryology laboratories that Dr. Dipti had brought up earlier. "You know what I don't like here?" she answered. "They don't pay the donors." I was surprised about this comment, as I had never come across such a complaint in the clinics where I conducted fieldwork. But Dr. Dipti suggested that the line between being a patient and being a donor in some IVF clinics may be porous. Her statement "they don't pay the donors" made sense, when the term "donors" was understood as patients providing "donor" gametes without their explicit knowledge. This concurred with rumors I had heard earlier, for instance, that the number of people undergoing embryo transfers would exceed the number of egg cell retrievals.

While "in other countries they can trace every single egg," as one clinician once remarked admiringly, in India there is no oversight through a national registry so far.[10] The number of eggs retrieved is noted down only in the clinic's laboratory records as well as the patient's prescription paper, or in some hospitals nowhere at all.

According to the rumors I heard from Dr. Dipti and several other interlocutors, some hospitals, particularly low-cost hospitals, may recruit donors from their own patient population by employing a rather wide interpretation of the term "leftover."[11] When patients indicate on informed consent forms that they agree to donate their gametes and embryos in case of any leftovers, they usually assume that "leftover" designates cells that they decide to donate *after* conception or even after the completion of their family. Clinicians, however, may understand those gametes (particularly egg cells) to be leftovers that exceed a certain quantity, for example the number of embryos that can be transferred in the current cycle. Rather than fertilizing all egg cells and cryopreserving the exceeding embryos, supernumerary eggs may be diverted to other patients. To put it in the words of an embryologist, in some clinics, "donation has priority over freezing." While the couples receiving donations would know about and pay money for their roles as recipients, it is said that most "donors" are not explicitly informed about and compensated for their "donation." To give a concrete example, if ten egg cells are retrieved from one woman, doctors would tell her that only five were recovered and directly divert the other five to the recipient. Since only five egg cells would appear on the "donor's" medical record, medical documents would be in order.[12] The ones who would lose out in these kinds of arrangements, however, are patients whose eggs are passed on and who would need them later. Minakshi, for instance, wondered why she did not have any leftover embryos after her first failed IVF attempt in a low-cost hospital. Her suspicion that her embryos might have been sold illustrates the anxieties prevalent in IVF hospitals: "They didn't freeze mine, that's the mistake they did. If they had frozen, it would have been quicker this time. Now we have to repeat the entire procedure. . . . There were five in total, three were inserted, and the remaining two were spoiled. I don't know if those were spoiled or not but they refused to freeze them. . . . They could do anything with the frozen embryos, I am sure they sell it to people who need them. If somebody benefits because of me, there is nothing wrong in it. But mine should also be successful."

What is striking about Dr. Dipti's critique as well as Minakshi's suspicion is that both were indignant not about the mixing of reproductive substances without patients' explicit consent but about the idea of doctors earning from these transactions and "donors" being left without any insurance in case their own cycle fails. Even though Dr. Dipti resented physicians for supposedly gaining economic profit without passing it on to donors, she justified mix-ups per se by referring to recipients' despair: "They need a child no matter what, they are desperate" (for the framing of infertile populations as desperate, see Franklin 1997). In this regard, it is important to note that most rumors of intentional redistribution concern low-cost hospitals in which patients in need of an egg donor could never afford to pay for a proper commercial donor. Redistribution would therefore ensure that the ones who also cannot revert to intrafamilial donors could still undergo third-party IVF cycles.

Stratified Sharing

The trope of distressed patients is also frequently invoked in low-cost hospitals in order to mobilize patients to *share* their egg cells. Egg sharing functions according to the same redistributory logic as depicted in the rumors: a certain number of eggs are assigned to a fellow patient. However, it involves the consent of both parties. It is considered to be a legitimate form of mixing and a frugal way to divide the costs for ovarian stimulation in order to make third-party cycles affordable to wider segments of the patient population. In this spirit, it is also encouraged by the *National Guidelines* (Government of India 2005, 68).

Many patients in low-cost hospitals agreed to egg sharing with the reasoning that their egg cells belong to the hospital anyway. "It is theirs [the doctors']," one of them remarked. "They have done everything. It is up to ma'am [the doctor in charge] . . . whatever the center feels is good for the eggs." In cases in which patients were reluctant, doctors sometimes complained. "They see all these people here in the waiting room and they know how they are suffering—how can they refuse to donate?" In contrast to high-cost hospitals where a couple's right to ownership over their gametes is emphasized, couples in low-cost hospitals are expected to generously share their reproductive substances. Physicians presume a community of suffering, in which patients are connected not only through a common medical condition but also through the boundless mixing of substances—a kind of involuntary "biosociality" (Rabinow 1996; for a discussion of biosociality in the Indian context, see Bharadwaj and Glasner 2009) or lateral "bioavailability" (Cohen 2005).

Moreover, similar to Marriott's (1968) description of transactions between caste groups, members of lower classes are expected not only to give but also to receive in an uncontrolled manner, as egg sharing implies that recipients cannot choose their donors. While middle-class patients are often very selective in terms of donor gametes, working-class patients are expected to accept substances from unknown sources and not to be affected by possible boundary transgressions. They are presumed to be ready recipients and are subjected to a gamete exchange system that they are not able to control. One could thus argue that Marriott's "model of stratified transactions" (170) regarding rank translates into a process of "stratified reproduction" (Colen 1995; see also Ginsburg and Rapp 1995) in terms of class.

An Age of Mix-Ups

The anxieties about mismatches and mix-ups presented here go beyond articulating discomfort with clinical practice. Relying on Jacob Copeman's (2013, 204) observation that substances have the ability "to form the basis of critique of the socio-political status quo," I argue that fears and rumors pertaining to gamete mixings may be read as larger moral panics in contemporary urban India, particularly harbored by the middle class.

The rise of rumors in different parts of the world has been interpreted by some anthropologists—in a rather broad-brushed manner—as an effect of "millennial capitalism and the culture of neoliberalism" (Comaroff and Comaroff 1999, 279). Rumors about the sale of body parts to be used for fertility potions, for example, have been widely circulating in contemporary South Africa. In his microsociological analysis of comparable rumors in Central and West Africa, Julien Bonhomme (2012, 226) shows that they all relate to the dangers of anonymity as "a key aspect of modernity." He argues astutely that these rumors are "not only new imaginings for new times, but also more precisely 'new imaginings for new relationships' (White 2000, 22)" (Bonhomme 2012, 226). As an epitome of "technological modernity" that enables interactions between strangers (205), IVF can similarly be interpreted to provoke rumors and fears, exactly because it substantially connects people who would not interact with each other in daily life.

Further, anonymity in the field of reproductive medicine evokes anxieties about uncontrolled and possibly inappropriate forms of mixing not only with people too distant but also with people too close. As demonstrated in the online comment above, incest is another specter haunting IVF (Porqueres i Gené and Wilgaux 2009; Wahlberg 2018). Many patients as well as clinicians worried that policies of anonymity with regard to gamete donations and the inadequacy of record keeping in IVF hospitals might lead to consanguineous relations in the future. Since 2005, the Indian Council of Medical Research has tried to curb these anxieties through guidelines and bills. But although the Assisted Reproductive Technology (Regulation) Bill of 2020 states that "[a] bank shall not supply the sperm or oocyte of a single donor to more than one commissioning couple" (Government of India 2020, 11), donors could still donate in multiple banks since, so far, there is no central registry in place that collects and matches data. "Sometimes I think we are doomed with this donor business," Dr. Nishika expressed her concerns. "Without even knowing, half-brothers and half-sisters might get married in the future." Dr. Nishika exhibited a dystopian vision of "doom" coming to reign through IVF—similar to *kaliyug*, the present age, which is described as a time of deterioration. *Kaliyug* denotes an age of distorted hierarchies and uncontrolled sexuality in which the observance of social and moral boundaries is in danger. An age in which "castes are mixed and all follow their own rules" (Tulsidas, as cited in Hess 1988, 245). An age of mix-ups, so to say.

Finally, fears and rumors about IVF mix-ups may not only exhibit anxieties regarding nonnormative forms of relatedness but also constitute a critique of the mixing of distinct social spheres that ideally should be kept separate: medicine and market. While "healing professions—including clinical medicine—in India have long been viewed as sacred, with medical/healing work looked on as noble and imbued with extreme religious merit" (Bharadwaj 2006, 461), a high number of doctors in Delhi mentioned that respect for their profession has been rapidly decreasing (for China, see Wahlberg 2018, 165). As Dr. Nishika explained, "A lot has changed. You know people used to revere doctors. They were next to god. Now that has changed and people don't trust. In fact lot of distress started because of malpractice. So people don't trust doctors as much as they used to." Diminishing trust may be connected to the privatization and corporatization of the Indian health care sector and the concomitant shift toward target- and profit-oriented medicine (Bharadwaj 2016, 238). This is reinforced by a legislative void in the case of IVF, allowing hospitals to operate with hardly any oversight. The fact that skepticism about the medical profession was widespread among patients *and* doctors may be another explanation for the prevalence of rumors about gamete mix-ups. According to my interlocutors, the mixing of medical care and economic profit constitutes a mismatch that might give rise to more substantial mix-ups.

Fears and rumors not only reveal prevailing reproductive norms as well as the perceived dangers of their transgression but also constitute sociopolitical commentaries on an age of mix-ups. More specifically, they point to moral panics about new relations distorted by anonymity in contemporary urban India and provide a critique of profit orientation in a highly commercialized health care sector.

The advertisement for a sperm donor made clear that IVF is fraught with anxieties because of its capacity to establish substantial relations across social boundaries. Instead of prompting the celebration of new possibilities of relatedness, the technology rather evokes moral panics in a highly stratified society. Since reproductive substances are imbued with the power to connect, their movement through IVF hospitals elicits fears and rumors about possible mismatches and mix-ups. As seen in two examples of gamete mixing, patients and medical professionals navigate IVF as a potentially threatening (and sometimes promising) procedure because of its ability to establish ties with people too distant or too close.

Middle-class patients who use commercial third-party cycles manage the specter of adulteration through attempts to establish continuity and, most important, secrecy. They try to silence what they consider to be inappropriate relations in order to be able to acknowledge children conceived through donor gametes as their "own." While they are still able to exert some command over processes of mixing, working-class patients, on the other hand, are much more likely to be subjected to regimes of gamete circulation outside their control, considering rumors and practices of gamete sharing in IVF laboratories. These stratified forms of mixing once again illustrate the social inequalities with which IVF practice is imbued.

After examining the ability of substances to generate relations—whether desired or not—I now turn to the laboratory as a site where substances are themselves constituted relationally. This involves a change of scene: away from homes, consultation rooms, and counseling sessions to the more enclosed realms of the hospital and to people who often remain invisible.

INSIDE THE LABORATORY
Embryo Ethics

Dr. Dipti was watching the embryos assembled in a petri dish under her micro-scope.[1] She felt content: they had developed nicely. Tomorrow she would select the best ones and transfer them to the uterus of her patient. She stood up from the workstation to carry the petri dish back to the incubator where it would be stored until transfer. Suddenly, Dr. Dipti stumbled, the dish slipped out of her hands, and its contents spilled on the floor. This is the moment when Dr. Dipti would wake up, relieved. It was just another one of her nightmares. These dreams, in which she would lose embryos, continued to haunt her on a regular basis. They convey a sense of the laboratory as a space dominated by unpredictability. When dealing with embryos, embryologists constantly face a loss of control. Not because petri dishes fall (I never encountered an accident like this during fieldwork) but because gametes might not fertilize, embryos might not develop as expected, or they might not implant in the uterus. As one doc-tor remarked, "This is not math where two and two are four. This is biology, it changes every minute. We cannot predict things." While unpredictability is valued in experimental setups (Rheinberger 1994), it constitutes a disturbing factor in IVF hospitals where, as we have seen, signs in waiting rooms promise quite definite success rates.

Embryologists manage unpredictability by engaging with embryos in various ways. On the one hand, they try to control embryos, for example, by surveilling or manipulating them with medical technologies. Similar to Rayna Rapp's (1999, 192) account of chromosomes, embryos "are work objects that must be deeply

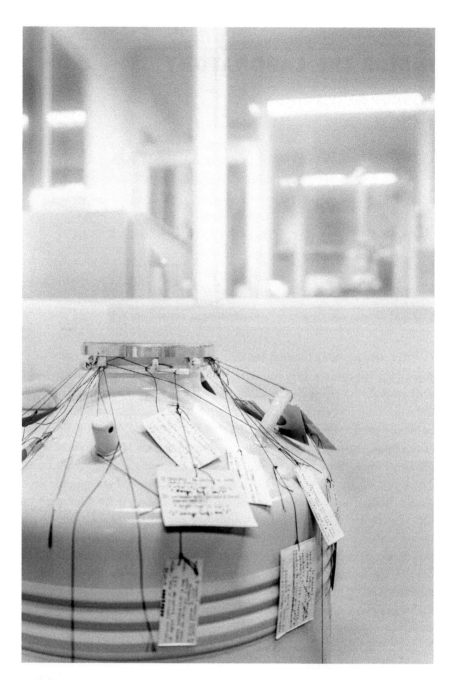

FIGURE 10. Cryopreservation tank in an embryology laboratory. Photo by Chhandak Pradhan.

and scientifically manipulated." In fact, embryos become viable only because they are shaped through laboratory practice. On the other hand, embryologists carefully tend and respond to biological substances. The laboratory environment is designed according to the perceived needs of embryos. And some embryologists understood their role in the laboratory not only in terms of following medical protocols but also in terms of themselves being responsive toward the embryos they are working with. "Sometimes when I am in the lab, according to the material, . . . I have to change my approach," Dr. Jaideep explained. In this sense, laboratory work resembles the ways in which clinicians work on and with bodies during the time of ovarian stimulation.

The fact that embryos remain indeterminate despite these efforts constitutes not only an epistemological but also an ethical challenge. Working with elusive substances that are neither clinical patients nor scientific research objects raises a host of questions for many embryologists. Dr. Rahul, a senior embryologist, therefore described embryology not only as a technical but also as an ethical task. "One's character has to be very sincere in doing embryology work." I address the ethical dimensions of laboratory practice relying on Michael Lambek's (2010) and Veena Das's (2012) notion of "ordinary ethics." As ordinary ethics do not necessarily manifest in dramatic decisions but are implicit in everyday clinical life, I argue that the clinical gaze is simultaneously an ethical gaze. Every time embryologists engage with embryos, not only their medical knowledge or technical skills but also their "ethical judgment" (Lambek 1997, 139) matters. Since ethical judgments vary, I analyze distinct forms of embryo ethics that permeate routine practice in embryology laboratories.

The Heart of the Clinic

The moments when I was able to visit embryology laboratories during my fieldwork always felt special to me. The laboratory of an IVF clinic is the place in which egg cells and sperm are handled after their retrieval from patients' bodies, fertilization takes place, and embryos are cultured in incubators until their transfer to the uterus.[2] It is one of the most protected spaces of the hospital—what some interlocutors called the "heart of the clinic."

Rarely in direct communication with patients, embryologists usually remain invisible in IVF clinics. They work either as freelancers visiting several clinics per month, or they are stationed in one hospital. Dr. Dipti once distinguished "three types" of embryologists, according to their educational qualifications: first, people who are medical doctors—for example, gynecologists who undertake additional embryology training, a group she herself belonged to and considered to be the crème de la crème of embryology. Embryologists in this category are highly sought after, and they often work as freelancers for several hospitals. The second group consists of scientists trained in biology, biotechnology, or biochemistry. Most of them attain their specific embryology skills either through a formal training program or an observership in an IVF hospital. The third group, at the bottom of the professional hierarchy, are people who start their careers as lab technicians and work their way up. Embryologists in this last group are often extremely dependent on the clinicians they work for.

Because the position of embryologists within the IVF world is quite vulnerable, at the time of my research professional associations started to be formed. "Embryologists don't have a forum right now. . . . As a body they don't exist," Dr. Rahul explained. "Anyone can take advantage of you in terms of making you do things. . . . If there is a body, there is one voice. We can all stand up and say, 'Sorry, we don't accept this.' This is what is required, otherwise we will not be able to protest." Many embryologists mentioned that they are under pressure to maintain high success rates. And, as one interlocutor put it, "the pressure of success . . . makes the unethical endemic." However, embryologists in India are not only situated within clinical hierarchies but also within broader regulatory structures. They are subjected to bioethical regimes in which embryo protection features quite prominently. The *National Guidelines* and the Assisted Reproductive Technology (Regulation) Bill are both modeled on British legislation and contain detailed rules about the handling of embryos. Yet, unlike their counterparts in the United Kingdom, embryologists in India are "not regulated persons," as Dr. Rahul put it, because there are still no *legally binding* frameworks. Nevertheless, most interlocutors understood themselves to work in ethical ways. Not necessarily because of their orientation to "transcendental, objectively agreed upon values" as fixed in guidelines, "but rather through the cultivation of sensibilities *within* the everyday" (Das 2012, 134), as became apparent in routine laboratory life.

Embryo Culture

"What is embryology?" Dr. Jaideep, a senior embryologist in a low-cost private hospital in Delhi, asked me rhetorically in a conversation and answered his question in the same breath: "It is the culture of gametes and embryos." The term "culture" not only implies connotations of growth and development, but also of nurture and care. In order to develop, embryos require care, Dr. Jaideep continued to explain. "If we do not handle embryos nicely, then they will not give a pregnancy. . . . I think it is the same as a mother bringing up their children to that

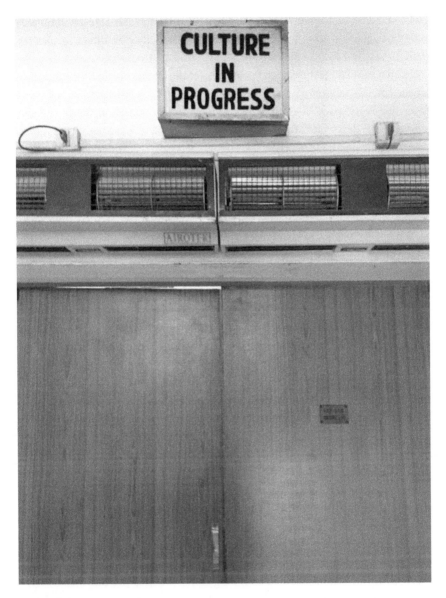

FIGURE 11.   Entrance to an embryology laboratory. Photo by the author.

stage. I bring the oocyte [egg cell] from the oocyte stage to the embryo stage."
Embryos require nurturing under very specific conditions between the point in
time of their generation in the laboratory (through the fertilization of gametes)
and their transfer to the uterus of the patient. And the best care, according to
embryologists, is to imitate in vivo conditions. "We try to mimic nature here,"

was a standard comment. "Nature," as imagined in the laboratory, is simulated with the help of an elaborate technical machinery including air filters, incubators, petri dishes, and culture media.

In vivo simulation starts with the location of the laboratory. In an ideal clinical layout, the IVF laboratory is located in a far-off corner of the hospital, removed from the hectic pace of clinical life.[3] Similar to the operation theater, people who enter undergo elaborate procedures of cleansing (e.g., changing of clothes, scrubbing of hands). But while the operation theater can be accessed by doctors, nurses, and patients, admission to the embryology laboratory is reserved for people working inside its bounds as well as senior doctors. The laboratory is also the only room with an air filtration system and positive pressure so as to reduce the risk of contaminants entering the room.

While restrictions of access and air filters regulate the environment of the room, incubators provide an emulation of in vivo conditions on a smaller scale. They are the machines in which petri dishes containing gametes and embryos are stored. Because they provide a specific microclimate for biological substances to develop (in terms of temperature, gas composition, and humidity), incubators are often compared to a uterus. Embryos are taken out of the incubator as briefly as possible so that they do "not get exposed to disturbed conditions and not get stressed for a long time," Dr. Dipti explained. When embryos have to be moved, the equipment used to transport them is prewarmed to simulate the temperature of the human body. Some embryologists even use their own bodies to keep embryos warm, for instance by covering the tip of the transfer catheter with their hand right before embryo transfer. Similarly with egg cells: during their retrieval, nurses hold the test tubes (in which the follicular fluid, which contains the egg cells, is collected) tightly in their fists. I once observed an embryologist scolding a nurse, when she delivered the tubes to him and he noticed her cold hands, with the words: "Your hands are cold, the eggs will die." Ideally, gametes and embryos should be moved not only as quickly but also as carefully as possible. Embryologists solved the tension between speed and caution in various ways. Some emphasized the importance of "finishing the job" as fast as possible, "like in a video game." Others highlighted their diligence. Dr. Dipti, who had the recurrent dream that a petri dish with embryos would slip her hands, always moved with the utmost caution.

Within the incubator, embryos are stored in petri dishes that contain a liquid—culture media—which supplies nutrients for embryonic growth.[4] Prepared by embryologists themselves until a couple of years ago, IVF culture media today is manufactured by specialized companies and sold through medical distributors, as a senior embryologist explained. "Media is more or less standard now. . . . There are two or three major players who are supplying media all over the world. So the same media is being used by me, by someone in America, or by someone in Australia. They [the manufacturers] are ruling the world right now." Most junior embryologists I talked to appreciated the turn to standardized and quality-controlled options for embryo culture. In their opinion, ready-made imported media was better than self-made media or media manufactured in India. "They [foreign companies] check whether it is embryo-safe and give the report, so we know," a junior embryologist remarked.[5] Some senior embryologists, on the other hand, lamented the disappearance of self-made media, not only because it was cheaper but also because, according to them, the rigid standards that media manufacturers impose are not necessarily compatible with biological processes. "These things are not chemistry but biology," Dr. Jaideep contended. "Human bodies vary, and all systems work differently, and biology adjusts itself to different environments. The new machines [he was referring to media and incubators alike] standardize everything." Although Dr. Jaideep was forced to use commercial media in his practice, he regularly subverted the company's usage instructions according to his own requirements. Embryology for Dr. Jaideep did not necessarily consist in executing standardized protocols in a technically sound manner but in working with and being responsive to biological material.

Whether adhering to standardized protocols or adjusting to embryos, laboratory practice is geared toward simulating the conditions of the human body. In order to culture embryos in vitro, embryologists employ machines and other medical equipment that supposedly model "nature."[6] However, they cannot fully succeed in this endeavor. "It is said that everything is suboptimal, if you compare it to human conditions," a doctor sighed. But embryologists do not always strive for an accurate model of the human body anyway: the advantage of IVF is exactly that it also provides possibilities of technical manipulation. And although embryologists carefully tend to the perceived needs of embryos, they simultaneously try to manipulate and control them.

Embryo Enhancement

Medical professionals often regard embryos of infertile couples as suspicious. Their quality is assumed to be "worse than normal." They might even be the reason why reproduction failed. Embryologists therefore attempt to improve the biological substances they are working with. They are "in pursuit of the perfect embryo," to quote the slogan of an embryology training course I attended. This implies that biologicals are not only embedded in relations that nurture them but simultaneously shape and enhance them.

Most of the enhancement techniques used in IVF laboratories consist of promoting or substituting reproductive processes: ICSI, assisted hatching, and embryo glue, to name just a few, are all supposed to mechanically advance fertilization, hatching, and implantation.[7] The most prominent enhancement technique is ICSI, which enables the direct injection of one single sperm into one egg cell instead of combining eggs and sperm in a petri dish and waiting for fertilization to happen on its own. Opinions among embryologists were divided about the appropriate degree of intervention. Should ICSI be conducted for every patient? Or only for patients for whom fertilization failures are expectable?[8] The proponents of "ICSI for all" argued that fertilization rates are better with ICSI, "since you yourself put it [the sperm] in the egg." Doctors were also worried that they "have to give some result" to their patients, who would blame them if fertilization failed. They further contended that rapidly increasing male fertility problems make ICSI imperative for more and more couples anyway, as "these kind of sperm will never make the way to the egg on their own." Others, however, argued that they only conduct ICSI when indicated (e.g., by low sperm quality) and preferred IVF over ICSI because the fertilizing sperm is selected "naturally." Even if ICSI was mandatory, some embryologists carefully selected the sperm cell used for injection by placing semen in one corner of a droplet and then choosing the cell that reached the opposite side the fastest. In this sense, they adhered to the idea of modeling "nature" even while employing enhancement techniques.

The use of enhancement techniques demonstrates that not only the lab environment but also reproductive substances themselves are technically managed. Embryos are shaped as entities adequate for IVF—namely, as entities capable of development and implantation. But still, embryos remain unpredictable: they often do not develop as expected or even at all. Embryologists therefore observe their growth in order to be able to select what they consider to be "good-quality" embryos for transfer to the uterus of the patient.

Embryo Selection

The advantage of IVF over other procedures in the field of reproductive medicine is described to patients as excorporating inner bodily processes. Along with the possibility of manipulation, this provides clinicians with the opportunity to visualize and observe embryos over time in order to make judgments regarding their quality. The entanglement of vision and knowledge has a long-standing history in biomedicine. Maurice Bloch (2008, S22) notes that the English term "evidence" etymologically stems from the Latin word *videre* (to see), which leads him to infer "a well-established European connection between seeing and truth." Similarly, Shigehisa Kuriyama (1999, 154) argues that epistemological discourses in biomedicine have long conflated seeing and knowing (see also Daston and Galison 2010; Foucault 1973; Hacking 1981). The process of IVF epitomizes this logic of visualization: it drags fertilization and embryonic development into the clinical limelight, transforming formerly hidden processes into observable ones with the promise to know. Embryologists follow the development of embryos through microscopes, judge their quality, and ultimately select the most promising for transfer.[9]

Aesthetic Assessments

While there are various methods of embryo selection, assessing the likelihood of reproductive success in distinct ways (e.g., genetic diagnosis, metabolic profiling, morphological analysis), most of them are too costly or technically unfeasible thus far.[10] In daily clinical life in India, embryo quality is for the most part evaluated according to morphological criteria—that is, the embryos' approximation to or deviation from aesthetic norms. This means that embryologists visually examine embryos under a microscope, evaluate them according to certain criteria, and classify them on an abstract scale. For instance, the higher the percentage of fragmentation, the lower the grade of the embryo. The assessment regarding form and developmental stage of the examined embryos simultaneously constitutes a process of selection, since only high-grade embryos are transferred to the uterus of the women or cryopreserved for further use.

While some embryologists only looked at embryos in the final stages of their development, others tracked them several times under the microscope in order to document their progressive growth. As one of them explained, "from the starting, oocyte [egg] quality and so play into it [embryo development] and one should observe that. It is like the difference between planned cultivation and wild cultivation, where planned cultivation means good work." In order to trace single embryos over time, some embryologists used droplet culture, where each embryo occupies its own drop of culture medium and can thus be tracked individually.

The necessity of visualization, however, conflicts with the requirement to avoid removing embryos from the incubator. Most embryologists could therefore only take a few glances at embryos during their development. They also had to decide within seconds which of the embryos to transfer. This situation might change with a technology that entered the Indian market in 2012: the "Embryo-Scope," a device developed by a Danish company. Since it aptly illustrates one way in which embryologists deal with the epistemological challenges they face in the laboratory, I describe the machine in detail.

Extensive Surveillance

"What do your embryos do when you sleep?" Dinesh posed this question to potential customers at a conference of fertility experts in Delhi. The director of a medical distributor company, Dinesh had recently incorporated the Embryo-Scope into his company's product line. Even though the EmbryoScope had found its way to only a few clinics in India so far, distributor companies had started to advertise it heavily, fertility professionals debated its usefulness, and more and more hospitals considered adding it to their technological setup.[11]

The EmbryoScope is essentially an incubator with an integrated camera that takes pictures of each stored embryo at regular intervals to visualize embryonic growth. It situates embryos within a close-knit net of surveillance and provides "systematic data on how embryos behave" over time, as Dinesh formulated it. The EmbryoScope reduces the need for direct engagement and even provides a means for collective decision-making: embryologists and clinicians can select their favorites on any computer screen. Since the pictures are saved, the EmbryoScope also enables the creation of an archive of images and data so that a specific embryo can be compared to previous exemplars. This might lead to the introduction of new indicators of embryo viability and provoke a reconsideration of current standards. The EmbryoScope thus addresses the concrete epistemological problems embryologists face in the laboratory in a specific way: it offers a dynamic gaze to capture the kinetics of developing embryos through time-lapse images. Still based on the premise of selection according to morphological criteria, the EmbryoScope embodies the modern idea to see "farther, better, and beyond the human eye" (Sturken and Cartwright 2009, 281). Within the logic of the EmbryoScope, closer surveillance equals better access to embryos.

Despite the extensive surveillance and concomitant "datafication" (Ruckenstein and Schüll 2017; see also van de Wiel 2019) the EmbryoScope offers, many embryologists experienced the morphological assessment of embryos as too detached. According to my interlocutors, surveillance—no matter how extensive—still implied a distance from the qualities embodied in biological substances. "We cannot tell which of the embryos will implant by just looking at them," was a common regret articulated by embryologists (Franklin 2006). This points to the fact that although there arguably exists a linkage between morphological features and implantation potential of embryos (e.g., Boiso, Vega, and Edwards 2002), the correlation of aesthetic values in the laboratory and clinical values in

terms of pregnancy rates is perceived to be far from certain by medical practitioners: embryonic beauty does not inevitably translate into clinical success. Thus,
embryos remain indeterminate despite clinical protocols and medical technologies aimed at their manipulation and visualization. This "routinization of
uncertainty" (Street 2014, 90) raises not only epistemological questions but also
ethical ones, especially in the context of embryo disposal.

Embryo Disposal

Once seemingly "good-quality" embryos have been transferred to the uterus
of a patient, the question arises of what to do with the other, so-called leftover
embryos: Should they be cryopreserved? Donated? Or disposed of? Embryo disposal constitutes one of the most contested realms of reproductive medicine,
especially in Euro-American, Christian contexts. Catholic moral philosophers,
for instance, employ the "potentiality principle" to oppose disposals as killings.
Embryos are precious human life, they argue, since "they possess the attributes
that they will have later in life" (Morgan 2013, S15). If the potential for personhood is ascribed to embryos starting right from the time of fertilization,
embryo disposal becomes a subject of fierce debate (for the notion of "saving,"
see Cromer 2018). However, the fact that embryo disposal does *not* constitute
a contentious decision in most embryology laboratories in India attests to the
diversity of embryo ethics. In daily laboratory life in India I encountered two
distinct ethical positions that permeate routine practice: life ethics and relational
ethics.

Existence: It Is Already Life

In contrast to Euro-American contexts, there is no prominent right-to-life movement in India, and embryologists in Delhi rarely ever have to position themselves vis-à-vis a pro-life stance. Dr. Pravin, for instance, could comfortably
acknowledge the variety of forms biological substances can take: "As far as I am
concerned, tissue is life, but it differs from person to person and lab to lab." I nevertheless met a few embryologists, all of them Christian, to whom questions of
life proved to be central. This is exemplified by the following sentence from an
informed consent form that was used in the IVF center of a Christian hospital,
run by the Church of India: "We [the couples undergoing treatment] also agree
to transfer the unused frozen embryos into my/ my wife's uterus without any
hormonal support essential for the successful outcome, if we do not wish to have
further pregnancy." This means that first, all leftover embryos were automatically

frozen in this hospital, and second, that they could *not* be discarded in case they were not needed by the couple anymore. The consent form stipulated that after their actual treatment was over, couples would have to return to the clinic, so that the unused embryos can be transferred to the uterus of the woman. Thus, the dilemma posed by leftover embryos was circumvented by returning embryos to the uterus of the female patient in the hope that they will *not* implant. Dr. Timothy, the doctor in charge of the unit, justified this rule with the explanation that reproductive procedures that are unacceptable to Christian faith are not permitted by the hospital. When asked whether a transfer without hope of implantation would not count as an act of disposal as well, Dr. Timothy shrugged: "Yes, in a way, but so many embryos are discarded in the uterus and go off." According to him, most patients used their frozen embryos in future cycles or renewed their storage contracts. In case patients stopped paying the cryopreservation fees, the embryos nevertheless remained in storage, and the hospital recorded the pending dues in the hope that patients would eventually return to provide their uterus for embryo disposal.

However, the question of embryo disposal was contested within the hospital. Isabel, the junior embryologist of the hospital and a Jehovah's Witness, found the thought of disposal through transfer highly problematic and wondered why the hospital did not start an embryo "adoption program." Since fertilized egg cells constituted human life for Isabel, discarding them (even via the uterus) equaled an abortion. Isabel was one of the few interlocutors who had thought about this topic extensively and identified the beginning of life with fertilization: "It starts with fertilization, when the chromosomes of the father and the mother join," she explained to me. "One does not expect an egg to form into an embryo and a living being, but a fertilized egg . . . yes. That's why it is already life." And once life had been created through fertilization, it shouldn't be destroyed. Her opposition to the hospital's embryo disposal policy was one reason why Isabel only worked with semen and had no ambitions to engage with embryos in the future.

The second example is Dr. Shila, an embryologist who was employed in a private hospital with predominantly Hindu staff. Dr. Shila was raised as a Hindu but converted to Christianity more than ten years ago (after she had already started her work in the hospital). She clearly distinguished between her personal life as a devout Methodist and her professional life as a scientist subordinate to clinicians' decisions. "It is a worldly work," she remarked about her occupation, "and has nothing to do with spirituality. I do this for being able to live." However, she always felt guilty when she had to discard leftover embryos, but "you have no choice, if patients don't make the payment [for cryopreservation]." Yet, although—as a good modern (Latour 1993)—Dr. Shila clearly distinguished between her professional handling and private valuation of embryos, or between worldly work and spiritual life, this distinction proved to be untenable. Her reluctance to discard embryos did play out in her practice more than she was prepared to admit. At least her colleagues used to mock her that she would always assign good grades to embryos (high-grade leftover embryos are usually frozen rather than discarded), which delayed the act of disposal until patients stopped paying for storage.

Although deliberations about fertilization as the beginning of life as well as the resulting ethical conundrums in clinical practice were not prominent in IVF clinics in Delhi, to Isabel and Dr. Shila embryos mattered because they constitute human life with an inherent potential for personhood. Isabel rejected the hospital's guidelines regarding leftover embryos and, as a consequence, refused to directly work with embryos. Dr. Shila was more agnostic when it came to practical cooperation within the hospital. But a few years after my fieldwork, she eventually quit her job as an embryologist to devote her life to more spiritual matters.

Becoming: Providing Bodies for Souls

Apart from these few examples, "life ethics" (Roberts 2007) were of no particular concern to most of my interlocutors, as one clinician explained in response to my probing. "To be very honest, I never thought about it. I thought it is part of my job, to put the patients through the treatment. The idea is to give them happiness that they conceive. That is my focus. Beginning of life and this philosophy, I never thought about it." Yet, laboratory staff nevertheless engaged with embryos in terms of life. To most of them it was crystal clear that embryos constitute biological life and therefore deserve care. "Of course, embryos are living entities, they develop," another embryologist remarked. But they just as well deserve care because couples had paid a considerable amount of money to create them. For instance, in case accidents happened in the laboratory (e.g., very rarely embryos got lost when they were transferred from one dish to the next during cryopreservation or thawing), embryologists were not so much concerned about the loss of life but about the economic damage for patients. As one of them explained, "Whenever there is a failure, it is not so much that 'oh, the embryo got destroyed' but it is more that 'the money we spent is gone.'"[12] Hence, life ethics constitutes just one way in which medical professionals relate to embryos.

In her fascinating study about IVF in Ecuador, Elizabeth Roberts (2007) points to the particularity of "life ethics" and describes another mode of engagement with embryos that she refers to as "kin ethics." In contrast to Ecuador's coastal areas, embryos in the Andes are perceived not so much as potential life by IVF practitioners and patients, but as future kin. In order to prevent their inappropriate circulation outside kinship circles, it is ethically imperative to destroy rather than cryopreserve them. This points to a valuation of embryos through concrete relations. Similarly in India, many interlocutors stressed what I call "relational ethics," with an added temporal dynamic: embryos grow in importance over time. Building on the work of scholars who note the fluid notions of personhood in different parts of India (e.g., Daniel 1984; Marriott 1968, 1976, 1990), Sarah Lamb (1997, 279) explores the "evolving nature of personhood conceptions over the life course." In the village in West Bengal where she conducted fieldwork, persons are conceived of as "inherently relational, each person functioning as a nexus within a 'net' (*jāl*) of ties shared with people (especially kin), places, and things." The number and intensity of these "substantial-emotional bonds" (283), which make up people, change over time: they increase over the life course and are supposed to decrease in old age. In a similar way, over the course of their development embryos are made up and come to matter through various relations.

First, for an embryo to count at all, it has to develop appropriately after fertilization. Similar to the time after embryo transfer, the few days when embryos are cultured in the laboratory are regarded by embryologists as a delicate time frame. While, as we have seen, they try to provide the most suitable technical conditions for embryos to develop, "in the end," many stated, "everything remains in god's hand." They explained that they only work as helpers or intermediaries. One embryologist, for example, dedicated his introductory textbook on embryology to "Mata Vaishno Devi who does everything at our center." In a few laboratories, I saw that doctors had placed gods in the form of small statues (*mūrti*) on their incubators in order to facilitate embryonic development. The time of development is thus considered to be a precarious stage, dependent not only on technical support but also divine intervention. Failure of the procedure—although tragic for patients—is not, however, interpreted in terms of a loss of life. Dr. Sajiv, for instance, explained that there is no "beginning of life" or a certain point in time when classifications switch from matter to life; rather, he continued, "the soul is permanent and there is no beginning." And when souls and bodies meet in the embryology lab, their specific destiny together could be very short-lived. While defining embryology as "providing bodies for souls," Dr. Sajiv was, however, wary about the quality of souls in his laboratory, as he did not want to be responsible for "bad people" populating the earth in the future. He therefore used to continuously play the *gāyatrī mantra*, in order to keep out of the room unwelcome souls, who may linger around waiting for a rebirth.[13]

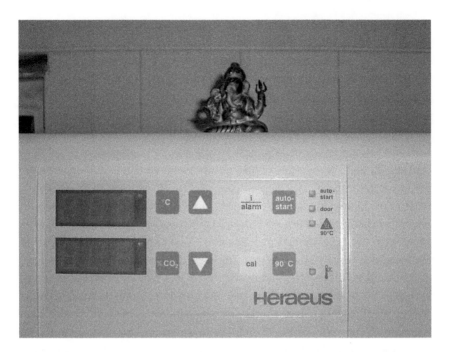

FIGURE 12.   Lord Ganesha on an incubator. Photo by the author.

Second, the "delicate dialogue between embryo and uterus," as one doctor put it, has to be successful, and implantation has to occur. "There isn't a huge issue with discarding embryos. Till an embryo implants, we don't really think that it is life. Because there are so many eggs which come out, so many embryos which are produced, so many of the embryos are discarded. Because when we are choosing embryos, selecting them based on morphology, so many embryos are discarded. And the embryos we are transferring, we don't know whether those embryos will implant or not. Therefore we don't take them very seriously till they implant." For many embryologists, an embryo turns into an entity that matters only after implantation. This is reflected in laboratory practice in which low-grade embryos are not considered worth saving, as they are unlikely to implant. They are sometimes used as practice material for junior embryologists or discarded. To give but one example, Dr. Kaushik one day encouraged me to have a look at the contents of a petri dish through a microscope: I could see an embryo in the middle of the plate. He then carefully removed the dish from the microscope stand and suddenly poured the contents into the dustbin. "It is an embryo that we cannot use anymore. It is not worth preserving. . . . I wanted to show you this. This is also part of IVF." Dr. Kaushik was of course aware of prevalent ethical debates in Euro-American contexts and wanted to educate me about the different manner in which he valued embryos.

Instead of development and implantation, some interlocutors identified the birth of a child as a significant event, particularly since IVF patients have a slightly higher risk of miscarriage during pregnancy. "For us a healthy baby born is really life," one clinician mentioned. "That is what . . . is success, that is what a parent can enjoy, that is what as a doctor I have done, that I can feel satisfied. Not just getting an embryo, just getting a positive pregnancy test. I don't consider all that." A colleague of hers also pointed out that fetal reductions are not uncommon among IVF patients (i.e., when more embryos than the desired number of children implant, selective abortions may be performed): "You must remember that in India the medical termination of pregnancy is legal [until week twenty]. So that is very practical. If you don't want a child, you can terminate it. [Patients] don't think of it as a living thing being destroyed. . . . But if there is a loss of a fetus, like she conceives and miscarries, that is very traumatic. 'Cause they have seen the fetal heart, they have seen the baby over there [on the ultrasound screen], and then they lose it. That is very traumatic for all of them." Hence, there is a clear differentiation between embryos to whom patients relate and those to whom they do not. This is also reflected linguistically: when patients sometimes consulted PremiumIVF for abortions, doctors would refer to the fetus as a "product." In contrast, when pregnant patients visited for prenatal care, they employed the terms "fetus," "embryo," or "child." In this sense, embryos come to matter only once they are recognized as future family members. And their importance manifests itself gradually, for example when the positive line appears on the pregnancy test or when the embryo's cardiac activity presents itself on the ultrasound screen.[14] The increasingly obvious manifestation of embryos over the course of a pregnancy is vital for their valuation as entities that matter.

This means that most of my interlocutors did not value embryos because of a potential that manifests when two gametes merge, but because of their relations once they develop and are connected to the uterus, the mother, or the family. Instead of an inherent potentiality, as in life ethics, what counts in relational ethics is gradually evolving relations. This also explains the fact that embryologists often told me about patients who forget about their frozen embryos once they conceive. "There are so many patients who make a cryopreservation payment, and then we never hear from them, never," a senior embryologist said. "They forget about it, they are least bothered about it." Once embryos have lost their relational potential to patients, they are simply not valued anymore.

As Dr. Dipti's nightmares indicated, embryologists constantly confront situations of unpredictability. Despite clinical protocols and medical technologies that pursue their manipulation and visualization, embryos continue to remain elusive. Embryologists, however, attempt to minimize failure by being responsive to embryos' perceived needs while simultaneously fashioning them as medically suitable and ethically acceptable entities. In a way similar to clinicians' relations to patients' bodies, embryologists work with and on embryos in conjunction with technologies, protocols, guidelines, and gods. Embryos as "matter related" (Abrahamsson et al. 2015) are thus constituted by various sociotechnical relations that they, in turn, shape.

Interpreting Dr. Dipti's dream further, one could argue that her apprehensions demonstrate not only the responsiveness but also the responsibility with which many embryologists engage with embryos in the laboratory. Embryologists' ethical gaze, in particular their judgment of embryos either as living beings or as relational entities, as it became discernable in clinical practice, matters in this regard. While in the former case, embryo disposal turns into a problematic issue in need of regulation, in the latter case it rarely elicits ethical attention. The notion of a dynamic set of relations through which embryos are constituted and sustained reveals a fluid understanding of biologicals: in terms of a process of becoming rather than a form of existence. And, one could argue, this constitutes a position equipped to deal quite pragmatically with unpredictability as a central epistemological experience in the laboratory. In contrast to different parts of the world where embryos often count as "icons of life" (Morgan 2009), and in contrast to distinct biological substances in India, such as blood (Copeman and Banerjee 2019), most embryos in Delhi's IVF hospitals remain surprisingly apolitical, reminding us that biological substances are always made through and situated within very specific sociopolitical, technological, legislative, and ethical relations.

Epilogue

In September 2016, the India Expo Centre in Greater Noida, located to the east of Delhi and part of the National Capital Region, was bustling with activity. Clinicians, embryologists, medical representatives, and an anthropologist all gathered at the convention center to attend a conference. Participants squeezed through the crowds in the corridors in their attempt to reach panels, which featured presentations of various disciplines: from endocrinology to embryology, from genetics to gynecology. Cordial greetings were exchanged here and there between colleagues who practice in different countries or just across the street.

Although conferences are frequently occurring events, this one was special. It was the 22nd World Congress of the International Federation of Fertility Societies. The fact that it took place in Delhi signaled that India had become part of a global conversation: not only as the surrogacy destination portrayed in international media, but also as an academic destination. Consider the contrast with Kolkata in the 1970s: a place where researchers like Dr. Subhas struggled to conduct IVF experiments, and a place from which a European company exported raw material. In a striking twist of medical history, hCG and other fertility drugs have since been sold back to India. Even more so, some stalls in the exhibition hall at Delhi's World Congress were occupied by Indian pharmaceutical companies that now produce these drugs locally.[1] Almost forty years after the world's first successful IVF procedure, it seems that India has made a mark in the world of reproductive medicine.

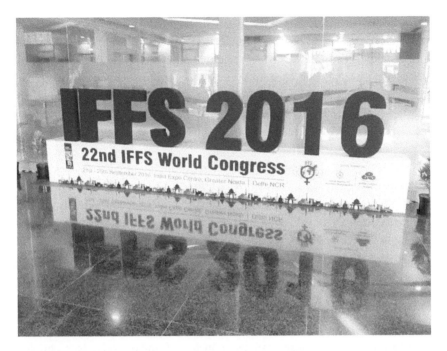

FIGURE 13. Entrance to the 22nd World Congress of the International Federation of Fertility Societies. Photo by the author.

In the first part of this book, I laid out the conditions of possibility for this event. I traced the genealogy of India's role in shaping global reproductive medicine from the 1960s up to the present day through three critical moments: the commodity chain of hCG from the subcontinent to Europe between the 1960s and 1990s, contestations around the first IVF experiments in the country between the 1970s and 2000s, and the emergence of a transnational IVF sector in Delhi since the late 1980s. I followed the travels of biological material, knowledge claims, medical supplies, and financial investments as vital parts that have animated global reproductive medicine. The three moments revealed how India has shaped global reproductive medicine throughout its postcolonial history in various ways: from a provider of raw material to a producer of knowledge and, subsequently, a thriving medical market.

Building on excellent accounts about the uses of IVF in different parts of the world, my goal was to demonstrate how a specific site, which is often relegated to the provincial, has had a share in the *making* of global reproductive medicine. I was interested to see what happens when we go beyond narratives of diffusion and instead examine India's role in the historical formation of this medical field. In what ways does global reproductive medicine emerge from a particular locale?

How can we tell a history of reproductive medicine through India without falling into the trap of nationalistic glorification? And what are the transnational interdependencies and asymmetries that make the history of IVF an interconnected but unequal one? These queries lead to a shift in analytical perspective: from questions around the use of IVF to a concern about its making. Rather than viewing IVF in India as an application of knowledge produced in other parts of the world, I highlighted India's variegated entanglements with global reproductive medicine.

In addition to India forming global reproductive medicine, this medical field itself has long informed the country's history. Populations became central targets for state interventions in the subcontinent as early as the nineteenth century. Shortly after Independence, the Indian government implemented a family planning program in the name of economic development and poverty alleviation (Sur 2017). Infertility, however, long remained in the shadows of population control efforts. This changed only in the late twentieth century, owing to a paradigm shift regarding the importance of comprehensive reproductive care, the technologization and standardization of infertility interventions, and, most important, IVF's economic profitability. In addition to population control, the health care sector in general and reproductive technologies in particular could now also be conceptualized as an impetus for economic development (Hodges 2013a). Once IVF had started to become a capitalist success, it could proudly be celebrated as part of the country's globalized modernity and be used to mobilize an image of India not only as a health care but also an investment destination.

Even though IVF in India has indeed turned into a financial opportunity for various actors, it is important to note that gains are distributed unequally. Stories about IVF's immense economic productivity mask the unavailability and unaffordability of services to most people. According to WHO estimates, there still is a "silent population of more than 180 million couples facing consequences of infertility" (Ombelet 2015, 106) worldwide. Countries in the global South are often disproportionately affected, as the lack of adequate primary and secondary health care may increase the risk of infertility. Despite current efforts in India to broaden the use of interventions in the tertiary sector (e.g., opening specialized public units), the IVF landscape is deeply inflected by asymmetric power relations: not only is access stratified, but medical practice differs between hospitals, and biological substances are handled according to patients' economic status. Thus, more often than not, the practice of IVF further reproduces entrenched hierarchies and aids in cementing social inequalities.

After analyzing the formation of reproductive medicine in India historically, in the second part of the book I examined its *contemporary making*. Entering hospitals and laboratories in Delhi, I tracked how various actors make IVF work as a delicate "ontological choreography" (Thompson 2005). Making IVF work means working on and with reproductive substances in conjunction with technologies, pharmaceuticals, protocols, and guidelines. Clinicians attempt to turn bodies designated as infertile into productive entities, make acceptable gametes that are understood to be improper, and manipulate embryos considered to be unpredictable. Following substances as they transform, travel, or simply elude us in IVF clinics served as a fruitful analytical tool to interlink intimate bodily processes and daily clinical life in hospitals and laboratories in India with larger social and ethical concerns.

The focus on mundane medical practice threw light on the substantial relations that reproductive medicine generates: between parents and offspring, donors and recipients, professionals and biologicals. I detailed the various kinds of connections, from the clinical to the commercial, from the epistemic to the ethical, which are summoned in daily clinical practice. While biologicals carry relational potential, they in turn are "matter related" (Abrahamsson et al. 2015). Interrogating how biological substances are constituted relationally, I tried to balance the tension of pointing to the vitality of substances on the one hand and their formation through often asymmetrical relations on the other. Although biologicals demand responsiveness and responsibility from clinicians, they are simultaneously fashioned as medically viable and ethically valuable entities for IVF.

The second part of the book further showed that as well as being a "hope technology" (Franklin 1997), IVF could simultaneously be described as a technology of discontent. Experiences of failure, fear, and unpredictability are prevalent in IVF hospitals. A sense of unease prevails when success is far from guaranteed, gametes travel uncontrollably, and medical practice demands ethically dicey decisions. This suggests that medical technologies are "unruly" (Mol 2008, 50). "[T]hey have an excess of, sometimes unexpected, effects" (47). Similar to other technologies, IVF might bring in its wake even more unintended consequences, whose reverberations may only become apparent over time. These anxieties are certainly reinforced by the legislative void that still characterizes India's IVF landscape.

However, global reproductive medicine in India as a complex, multiscalar, and ever-shifting assemblage will continue to change in the future. Take for example the passing of the Surrogacy (Regulation) Bill, 2019, by the Lok Sabha, which may start to regulate the commercial surrogacy sector in the future. Whether this is going to lead to shifts of commercial surrogacy procedures to the black market—as many commentators fear—or the relocation of the industry to neighboring countries, as has happened before (Deomampo 2016), or a complete standstill, remains to be seen. Should the Assisted Reproductive Technology (Regulation) Bill, 2020, become law, which would comprehensively regulate all IVF procedures, even more questions about IVF's future in India will arise. Or take another scenario: although IVF already oscillates between an exclusive, high-cost intervention and a low-cost alternative, it might further diversify. Global efforts to develop affordable forms (e.g., see Ombelet 2007) might extend the coverage of infertility care to a large degree. The spread of reproductive technologies beyond megacities has already become a reality. But what will it mean for the majority of India's population, who still cannot pay for the procedure, if IVF becomes accessible? What would IVF in its "fourth phase" look like? And how might such changes translate to medical contexts in the global North that are severely affected by austerity measures?

Global reproductive medicine in India will continue to shift in form and scope. With novel political or medical formations, reproductive medicine is going to not only reproduce but also reinvent itself. Observing and thinking through these mutations will be instructive for our understanding of various substantial relations in India and on a global scale.

Notes

INTRODUCTION

1. All names used in this book are pseudonyms, except for well-known people whose names are already in the public domain.

2. Although I mainly focus on IVF and ICSI (intracytoplasmic sperm injection) in this book, I use the terms "reproductive technologies" or "reproductive medicine" as more encompassing notions.

3. For a detailed overview, see Inhorn and Birenbaum-Carmeli 2008 or Thompson 2005.

4. Kahn 2000; Franklin 1997; Franklin and Ragoné 1998; Strathern 1992; Thompson 2005.

5. See, for example, Bharadwaj 2016; Birenbaum-Carmeli and Inhorn 2009; Inhorn and van Balen 2002; Knecht, Klotz, and Beck 2012.

6. Following Jean Comaroff and John Comaroff (2012), I use the term "global South" not in a substantive but in a relational sense that "always points to an 'ex-centric' location, an elsewhere to mainstream Euro-America, an outside to its hegemonic centers, real or imagined."

7. Abbasi-Shavazi et al. 2008; Bharadwaj 2002, 2003, 2006, 2016; Bharadwaj and Glasner 2009; M. Clarke 2009; Handwerker 2002; Inhorn 2003a, 2003b, 2004, 2006; Pashigian 2009; Roberts 2007, 2012; Wahlberg 2018.

8. To be precise, I include ICSI in my analysis, as it constitutes a routine procedure in many hospitals. The only difference to IVF is that eggs and sperm are not left in a petri dish to fertilize on their own, but one sperm cell is directly injected into an egg cell with the help of a micromanipulator.

9. While a snapshot invokes the image of a bounded surface (like a photograph), I imagine global reproductive medicine in India as a configuration that implies geographical width and historical depth.

10. See *Relative Values: Reconfiguring Kinship Studies*, in which "substance" is used to refer to information, rivers, and railways, or even family photographs (Carsten 2001, 29).

11. There are crucial nuances between reproductive substances. They differ in terms of their scarcity, renewability, detachability, transferability, convertibility, and mobility (Bärnreuther 2018). Further, they are often gendered and classed (Almeling 2007, 2011) and valued in various ways according to the contexts in which they move (Appadurai 1986).

12. In contrast to the dualism of substance and code or nature and law, as posited by David Schneider (1980), ethnosociologists have described "transactional thinking in South Asian society" as monist. This stance has rightly been critiqued as not only too simplistic but also orientalizing (Carsten 2001). Bracketing this question, I focus on the point relevant for my argument; namely, that flows of corporeal matter have been described to have substantial implications.

13. "[U]sing the tools . . . that have developed in more traditional anthropological studies . . . to explore the social dynamics of postcolonial technoscience" (Street 2014, 28–29) does not translate into the assumption that "India" or "biomedicine" "can be taken for granted as the context of people's actions"; rather, "[t]he power of the ethnographic

method lies in its capacity to locate universalizing projects such as biomedicine within their situated practices" (30).

14. The political-economic role of science and medicine in India has changed continuously over the decades: from a pillar of colonial oppression to a tool of nation-building and poverty alleviation in late colonial and postcolonial times to a driver of economic growth since the economic reforms in the 1990s (Hodges 2013a, 655; see also Arnold 2013).

15. This kind of cross-fertilization of family planning and infertility interventions was common in other areas as well: for example, laparoscopy, a surgical technique that was imported to India in the 1980s and initially used for tubal litigations, was later reappropriated by infertility specialists who employed it for the retrieval of egg cells.

16. I conducted fieldwork for six months in 2010, ten months in 2011–12, and five months in 2016 along with three stays of one month each in 2014, 2015, and 2017.

17. Laparoscopy is an endoscopic procedure used in IVF clinics to visualize the outside of the uterus, the fallopian tubes, and the ovaries to detect abnormalities. Hysteroscopy is used to inspect and/or operate on the inside of the uterus. Ovulation induction means ovarian stimulation with the help of hormonal medication to grow more than one follicle (which contain egg cells). This can be combined with intercourse, IUI, or IVF. IUI is a procedure where sperm is injected into the uterus of a patient. During an IVF/ICSI procedure egg cells are extracted from the body of the female patient, fertilized, and returned to the uterus of the patient or a surrogate mother, who carries and gives birth to the child.

18. I also conducted internships in two other IVF centers, which provided a valuable comparative perspective: one in a different state in India (2010) and one in Germany (2011).

19. Laura Nader (1972) coined the term in her call to research the powerful in the United States as part of a democratizing project. Even in the 1990s Hugh Gusterson (1997, 115) still remarks on their invisibility in ethnographies: "the cultural invisibility of the rich and powerful is as much a part of their privilege as their wealth and power, and a democratic anthropology should be working to reverse this invisibility."

20. In CommonCare I could more easily be placed in the scheme of things, since many PhD students of the college were doing research in different departments of the hospital.

21. Not all direct quotations in this book are verbatim, as they might be derived from notes typed out after interviews.

22. Similar to surrogacy, "[t]he terminology used to refer to the participants in [IVF] is diverse, contested, and often reflects a particular stance on assisted reproduction" (Deomampo 2016, 14). I decided to use the term "patient" rather than "IVF user," or "gamete donor" rather than "gamete provider," since it reflects the language of my interlocutors.

1. FROM URINE TO AMPOULE

1. Interestingly, urine itself has long been used as a transformative material, for instance for turning wool into garments, producing gunpowder, or tanning. But it was also a substance frequently employed in alchemy (Novick 2018).

2. The concept of a hormonal body or an "endocrine style of thought" (Gaudillière 2004, 525) in the life sciences and biomedicine is a relatively recent phenomenon. After the term "hormone" was coined in 1905 (Laveaga 2005, 744), most hormones as they are known today were scientifically described in the first half of the twentieth century.

3. "Since [gonadotropins] are proteins, not steroids, they could not be chemically synthesized" until the late 1980s when biotechnological methods became available (Sengoopta 2006, 203).

4. For the moral economy of academy-industry collaborations, see Nordlund 2015.

5. Born in Vienna, Bruno Lunenfeld fled to England and Palestine during the Second World War. After studying medicine at Geneva, he became interested in infertility for Zionist reasons (Livneh 2002; see also Novick 2018). Sometimes referred to as the "hormone pope," he has practiced, researched, and taught in various institutions, mainly in Israel.

6. Even though hMG is a different kind of gonadotropin, the processes and challenges involved in its industrial production are remarkably similar.

7. Unholy, because the Catholic Church later explicitly stated its opposition to many of the medical procedures which hMG has made possible. After Italy, the collection was extended to Argentina, Brazil, and Israel (Vertommen 2017).

8. Today, Moeders voor Moeders, owned by Aspen Pharma, still collects urine from pregnant women, "which Aspen Oss then processes into an active ingredient sold to the pharmaceutical company Merck Sharp & Dohme," which, in turn, had acquired Organon in 2007 (Kr-løkke 2018, 52, 59, 76). Between 1963 and 2006, Moeders voor Moeders also used to collect urine from postmenopausal women to produce hMG. The first collection sites were nunneries in Nordbrabant and Limburg (Moeders voor Moeders, n.d.a).

9. An interlocutor in India has made this brochure accessible to me.

10. This booklet is from the private collection of an interlocutor; it was printed around the mid-1990s.

11. The equity shares of Organon in Kolkata were divided between Organon (49 percent), the Mehta Group (49 percent), and a trust managed by nominees of Organon (2 percent), which effectively led to a constellation where "Holland was in control," as a former managing director said in an interview. I focus on Organon India since, to my knowledge, there was no other pharmaceutical company conducting similar urine collection programs in India.

12. The policy changes in India coincided with the reorganization of Organon's holding company, Akzo, in 1971. Organon was subdivided, and the manufacture and sale of bulk products outsourced to Diosynth, an independent "sister" (Tausk 1984, 172). Diosynth operated under the legal name of Organon in India until 1983, when it was "Indianized" after the permissible foreign equity share of MNCs had been limited to 40 percent under the Foreign Exchange Regulation Act. Organon (India) thus changed its name to Infar (India). According to my interlocutors in India, they used Infar's relative independence to initiate their own projects that were not necessarily related to international Organon strategies. Many employees in India strongly identified with the company and its unique work culture, the "Infar culture," a sentiment that is also reflected in the chorus of the "Infar Anthem": "Tera hai, Mera hai / Hum sab ka hai / Infar" (Inscape 2007, 37), which translates to "It is yours, it is mine / It is all ours / Infar." The company's name once again changed to Organon in 2002. For reasons of legibility, I refer to the company in India as Organon India, instead of Diosynth or Infar, in the remainder of the book.

13. According to Mr. Velden, one reason for this anxiety was that a newspaper in the Netherlands had published a report about the Dutch queen and her sisters using hCG for weight loss, even though Organon had not advertised this off-label use. Concerned that Dutch women might boycott the project, the company apparently decided to expand its operations to India. The Moeders voor Moeders website also mentions that a sharp decline in birth rates in the Netherlands in the early 1970s forced the company to extend its collection area to the whole country in order to keep the number of donors steady

(Moeders voor Moeders, n.d.a). This might have been connected to the introduction of the contraceptive pill in the 1960s.

14. Bodily excrements are often considered to be polluting substances in India, particularly excrements originating from social inferiors (e.g., Barrett 2008). Yet, interestingly, urine also counts as a powerful substance that "promotes strength, energy, fitness, and longevity" (Alter 2004, 185). Joseph Alter notes that in the context of auto-urine therapy "it is useful to think of one's own urine—as quite distinct from someone else's—as comparable to soma, as soma is understood in the medical literature to produce immortality by "killing off" the body prone to aging, disease, and death and replacing it with flawless reproduction" (192).

15. This concern was shared by lower-level workers employed for urine collection, such as collection boys or supervisors of collection centers. Mr. Roy, who was involved in the collection program as a worker, explained that he and his colleagues were similarly troubled about handling urine. But he stated that they got used to the substance after working with it on a daily basis.

16. According to my interlocutors, all low-level workers, such as ladyworkers and collection boys, were not formally employed by Organon India. They received monthly salaries as well as incentives for their work in cash through a subcontractor.

17. Bruno Lunenfeld similarly notes that menopausal women in Israel were not paid for donations because "they may add water to increase the volume" (cited in Vertommen 2017).

18. I thank David Arnold for suggesting this term in a discussion of an earlier version of this chapter during the workshop "Fringe Science and Threadbare Knowledge," held in Zürich in June 2017. For "corporeal magnanimity," see Simpson 2011, 255.

19. For the entanglement of family planning, poverty alleviation, and economic development, see Sur 2017.

20. This reasoning implies that women in India can decide to perform an abortion, if they find out that they are pregnant early on. The Medical Termination of Pregnancy Act from 1971 states that pregnancies may be terminated until twelve weeks by approval of one registered medical practitioner and until twenty weeks by approval of two registered medical practitioners. "The inclusion among the grounds for eligibility of failure of a contraceptive device made abortion more or less available on demand" (Rao 2004, 41).

21. In their application for a license, Organon had already stated that hCG "will be exported in full Qty" for an expected foreign exchange earning "in the order of Rs. 92,00,000/- for 5 years." The application further explained that "the unique feature of the project is that most of the production is planned to be exported due to its tremendous demand in international market" (National Archives of India 1977). The license was granted by the Government of India under the condition that Organon export at least 60 percent of the production of hCG to gain foreign exchange.

22. Jean-Paul Gaudillière (2005, 613) describes the importance of a "purification paradigm" in pharmaceutical culture. Within this paradigm, research and production strive for the preparation of "homogeneous (if not pure) compound."

23. The factory was sold to an Indian company, which still produces hormonal bulk drugs.

2. FROM DISMISSAL TO RECOGNITION

1. I refer to Dr. Subhas Mukherjee and Prof. Sunit Mukherjee by their first names, not only to avoid confusion because of their identical surnames, but also to reflect the language employed by most interlocutors.

2. Raina (1996, 169) also points out that, in this framework, reverse flows only consist of raw material or data.

3. This draft letter was part of Prof. Sunit's private collection containing official documents and letters of Dr. Subhas, which I consulted in 2014. It has since been transferred to the archives of the National Institute for Research in Reproductive Health.

4. This letter was also part of Prof. Sunit's private collection.

5. Among them were the 5th International Congress on Hormonal Steroids in New Delhi in November 1978, the satellite symposium of the congress in Varanasi, and the Indian Science Congress in Hyderabad in 1979. He also gave lectures at Gangaram Hospital in New Delhi and Gauhati Medical College (Anand Kumar 1997a, 528).

6. The history section disappeared from the various versions of the Assisted Reproductive Technology (Regulation) Bill.

7. More recently, the contribution of the embryologist Jean Purdy in the United Kingdom has also been recognized.

8. For many, Dr. Anand Kumar's words gained even more gravity, since by supporting Dr. Subhas's claim he lost his own status of having produced India's first IVF baby.

9. According to Prof. Sunit, the responsible gynecologist had initiated the media announcement without Dr. Subhas's consent.

10. In the United Kingdom, Dr. Robert G. Edwards faced similar challenges. On June 18, 1997, he explained in a letter to Dr. Anand Kumar, "As we worked in the early stages of IVF, all our grants were withdrawn by the granting authorities. I was ostracized in some scientific meetings, and we had to defend ourselves in the media from Popes, Archbishops, clerics, politicians, and the rest. Many scientists came to our labs to tell us to stop working on human embryos" (Churchill Archives Centre, n.d.).

11. They explained that, in the same way as crabs trapped in a basket prevent each other from climbing out (by pulling more advanced crabs downward), Dr. Subhas's colleagues prevented him from receiving recognition. A recent documentary on Dr. Subhas by Rajib Sarkar is titled *Effect of Indian Crab Syndrome* (*Deccan Herald* 2014).

12. See Abraham (2006) for a discussion of the ideological reliance of modern nationalism in India on local knowledge, and Prakash (1999) for the long-lasting intimate relationship between science, colonialism, and nationalism.

13. Simultaneously, however, they emphasized their international connections with commonly acknowledged centers of innovation.

3. FROM HOBBY TO INDUSTRY

1. It is important to mention that Dr. Chakraborty had not only been running an IVF facility but also carried out research projects in cooperation with several universities. Upon his retirement at the age of ninety, he donated his institute to the Indian Council of Medical Research. This is likely the only instance when a formerly private hospital has been turned into a government facility.

2. One could even argue that until today, IVF has never completely lost its experimentality, as one clinician remarked: "IVF is not a very old branch, it's only around thirty years old, so we don't know the long-term effects."

3. Reproductive medicine derived from the agricultural sciences in the beginning of the twentieth century and has always maintained close connections to this field (A. Clarke 1998; Cooper 2008).

4. Bharadwaj (2016, 122) notes that in 2011, "duty on imported equipment that was once as high as 115 percent has fallen to 25 percent."

5. Set up in 1942 by the colonial state, the Bhore committee conducted a survey in British India on the status of the health care system. Its results as well as recommendations to increase the coverage of the country's health services were recorded in a report in 1946 (Qadeer 2013, 152). "While the Bhore committee had recommended that

12 per cent of total outlay must be earmarked for health, the figure never crossed 3 per cent" (Baru 2003, 4435).

6. As mentioned earlier, I use pseudonyms when I talk about doctors and patients whose names are not in the public domain. In these cases, I use only first names, since it reflects the conventions of the hospitals where I conducted fieldwork.

7. Many corporate hospitals have also started to expand to second-tier cities (Lefebvre 2010, 21), where health care is offered in a less luxurious style and at a cheaper level (Sarojini, Marwah, and Shenoi 2011), following "the government's announcement in 2008 of a 5-year tax holiday for setting up hospitals in Tier II and Tier III towns" (Chakravarthi 2010, 202).

8. Dr. Nishika, for example, reopened her own nursing home a few years after the shutdown.

9. "ESIS is a social security program established in 1952 for organized labor in factories with 10 or more employees, which is mandatory coverage for workers earning less than Rs. 15,000 a month (and covers their families and retirees), and which combines employer, employee, and government contributions. CGHS, introduced in 1954, covers government (e.g. railways, defense) employees, dependents, and retirees, and it is funded by a combination of employee and central government contributions" (Burns 2014, 106). However, some couples covered under these programs felt uncomfortable submitting their IVF bills to office administrators, as their colleagues would come to know about their infertility. One woman stated that she would only hand in her medical bills in case her IVF cycle was successful—which left her empty-handed in a double sense when her pregnancy test turned out to be negative.

10. In contrast to other states in India, government employees in Delhi are not allowed to practice privately.

4. THE CLINIC AND BEYOND

1. "Success rate" is a tricky term, as there are various ways to define success: it can mean a positive pregnancy test (which includes biochemical pregnancies and later miscarriages), a clinical pregnancy at a certain time during the pregnancy (usually before patients are referred to an obstetrics department), or live birth rates (after the birth of a child). Further, success rates may be calculated per treatment cycle, per egg cell retrieval, or per embryo transfer. Hospitals rarely make public how they arrive at these numbers.

2. My goal is to avoid stereotypical depictions related to reproduction in India and instead underline the idiosyncrasies of each story. However, the emphasis on the importance of fertility in the following is due to the fact that all my interview partners had learned to understand themselves as infertile and actively sought medical interventions (Wilson 2014).

3. While many patients mentioned that they would be fine with either a son or a daughter as long as they got pregnant, there was a considerable number of cases in which parents who already had a daughter undertook a second round of IVF to conceive again (unlike couples whose first child was a son).

4. Some doctors also reported that many patients would only require counseling regarding the "right timing," meaning the fertile days of the cycle.

5. The Practice Committee of the American Society for Reproductive Medicine estimates that "up to 30% of couples who are unable to conceive are diagnosed with unexplained infertility" (2006, S111).

6. IUI is a procedure where sperm is injected into the uterus of a patient.

7. It is also used during third-party cycles in which reproductive cycles of donors and recipients are aligned.

8. Clinics that conduct only a few IVF cycles per month usually employ freelancing embryologists to reduce costs.

9. Ultrasonography is a constant feature during IVF cycles: it is used for initial diagnostic assessment of reproductive organs, for monitoring follicular growth, as assistive equipment for oocyte retrieval as well as embryo transfer, and as a means to detect the fetus's heartbeat. As Dr. Nishika pointedly remarked, "The moment you walk into this clinic, you'll get an ultrasound done. We need that in order to see."

10. While the notion of productivity is central for IVF practice, what counts as being productive has changed over time: a few years ago many clinicians aimed at harvesting the largest number of eggs possible. But recently many doctors have started to increasingly place value on "sustainability." They aim for the production of fewer but high-quality egg cells. Furthermore, there is a shift toward "natural IVF," in which the one egg cell that grows in a regular cycle is taken out of the body to be fertilized, making the process of ovarian stimulation obsolete.

11. Most deliveries of IVF babies are, however, conducted by caesarean section, since they are considered to be "precious pregnancies."

12. The IVF users she interviewed contested the trope through the language of investment, because it takes into account the hard work and active stance of patients.

13. Destiny and *karma* were often referred to simultaneously. As Lawrence Babb explains, "misfortunes . . . may be seen in more than one light. They may be seen as simply 'fated,' as caused by witchcraft or ritual omissions of some kind, or they can be interpreted as the karmic consequences of past misdeeds" (1983, 171). These distinct "frames of reference" imply different grades of moral responsibility and different possibilities for corrective action (171–73).

14. Francis Zimmermann points out that scholars' belittlement of such statements as coping mechanisms or strategies employed by doctors to shuffle off responsibility for failure does not do justice to the "covert Sanskrit categories" (2014, 86) underlying these expressions. By tracing "conceptual genealogies of medical arguments" (87), Zimmermann argues that rather than stopgaps called on when "rational" explanations fail (see Bharadwaj's [2006] notion of clinical theodicies), these explanations translate Ayurvedic principles of therapeutic prognosis.

15. Interestingly, a lot of stories circulate in IVF clinics about patients who get pregnant while they are "on a break" from interventions. Reasons cited for this phenomenon are the decrease in stress when patients don't have to visit the hospital as well as positive side effects that may have resulted from earlier interventions (i.e., the ovarian tubes might have been flushed and enabled a pathway for the egg cells to reach the uterus).

16. Among these are multiple births, possible birth defects, infections, complications deriving from anesthesia, or ovarian hyperstimulation syndrome.

17. The notion "modes of somatic activity" is inspired by Gesa Lindemann's (2002) work on intensive care units in Germany and her deliberations about the body's distinctive activity as it is expressively realized in clinical interactions.

5. WHEN CELLS CIRCULATE

1. It is important to note that Marriott confines his analysis to Hindu transactions and relies on fieldwork data from villages in Uttar Pradesh, North India.

2. See also Böck and Rao 2000; Carsten 2004; M. Clarke 2008; J. Edwards 2000; Franklin 1997; Pande 2009; Ragoné 1994; Sahlins 2013; Strathern 1992; Viveiros de Castro 2009.

3. In general, embryo donation was distinguished from gamete donation, since it was rather likened to adoption.

4. Thomas Laqueur (2000, 81) explains that similarly in Europe, "there is no historical model for women's reproductive substances venturing forth . . . because motherhood has almost exclusively been construed as 'bearing' and not as begetting."

5. My observations are of course biased in the sense that I was not able to meet people who did *not* return to medical institutions because they had decided against using donor gametes.

6. A third option is egg sharing, which I describe in the second part of the chapter.

7. In case of commercial gamete donations, patients, hospitals, and donor agencies all work together to manage relations in a way that they can be eclipsed or even forgotten (Bärnreuther 2018).

8. See Tine Gammeltoft's work on spectral kinship.

9. See Roberts (2012) for an account of how clinicians in Ecuador use third-party IVF cycles to "improve" the genetic make-up of the population and to contribute to a process of "whitening the nation."

10. According to the Assisted Reproductive Technology (Regulation) Bill of 2020, banks will have to keep records of gametes for at least ten years, "upon the expiry of which the clinic and bank shall transfer the records to a central database of the National Registry" (Government of India 2020, 9).

11. This does not entirely coincide with the public/private distinction.

12. By asking for a signature on the informed consent form, clinicians nominally conform to the *National Guidelines*. In this sense, "the primary function of consent forms is to protect the practitioner from liability, not to protect the patient from injury or abuse" (Gupta 2011, 173; see also Bharadwaj and Glasner 2009).

6. INSIDE THE LABORATORY

1. "Embryo" as a medical term is widely used for such diverse forms as human egg cells after fertilization, zygotes, blastocysts, and fetuses, and the borders are blurred on both ends of the spectrum (Roberts 2007, 184). In the two hospitals where I conducted fieldwork, the term was colloquially employed to designate the cluster of cells between the fertilization of gametes and their transfer to the uterus of the patient.

2. Some clinics also had a separate andrology laboratory, which was used for semen analysis and preparation.

3. In practice, the separation of the laboratory from other areas was accomplished to different degrees: sometimes the lab was almost completely set apart from the operation theater, as the door remained closed and biological substances passed through a hatch. At other places the door that connected both spaces remained open to facilitate the traffic between operation theater and laboratory. Finally, in one exceptional case I observed, the laboratory instruments were placed at the edge of the operation theater (this, however, constituted a temporary solution as a new lab complex was under construction).

4. While until a few years ago there were different kinds of media employed to model the different stages of the embryo's journey from the ovaries through the fallopian tubes to the uterus, most embryologists today use "sequential media," a type of media that provides "the right nutrients at the right time."

5. They explained that they would only use "foreign media" for IVF procedures (and hence for the cultivation of eggs and embryos), whereas "Indian media" could safely be employed for work connected to semen preparations (e.g., for IUI), as semen is less demanding. The distinction between "imported equipment" and "Indian equipment" is also made by medical distributors.

6. Some embryologists raised this motto from a technological to a moral level by proclaiming that they would only conduct "natural" procedures, which they interpreted as reproduction between a married man and woman.

7. Whereas some of these measures had turned into routine procedures, the usefulness of others was hotly debated: for instance, while some laboratories performed assisted hatching for all their patients (a process where the cell wall of the embryo is thinned with a needle or laser before the transfer in order to facilitate the hatching process in utero), others only employed it in selected cases.

8. Some clinics found a compromise in conducting ICSI for half of the eggs, while leaving the rest for IVF.

9. Selection of embryos became a routine practice in IVF clinics with the advent of gonadotropins, which allowed the production of a high number of egg cells and led to a disparity between the number of eggs produced and the number of embryos transferred in one cycle.

10. To my knowledge, there were only a few hospitals in Delhi where preimplantation genetic screening had been established on a routine level during my fieldwork (for a study of preimplantation genetic diagnosis in the United Kingdom, see Franklin and Roberts 2006).

11. However, some embryologists remained skeptical about the device. Besides the remarkable costs, the high exposure to light was viewed as potentially harmful to embryos.

12. This concurs with silent agreements in some clinics that the embryos of patients who pay reduced fees may be treated as experimental material. "There are only few embryos which you can afford to experiment on: those of charitable patients who do not make a full payment," explained one embryologist. In this sense, embryos' preciousness depends on their owners' affluence rather than an inherent potentiality.

13. Hospitals in South Asia are known for housing the spirits of deceased persons who died an unfortunate death or whose mortuary rites were not performed properly (J. Parry 1994, 128). Not being able to move on, they cling to the world and disturb the living. See Parry (233) for the power of the *mantra* "to put any ghostly assailant to flight."

14. More and more hospitals have started to show patients pictures of their embryos before embryo transfer, which might antedate this manifestation.

EPILOGUE

1. One has to note, however, that Indian pharmaceutical companies engaged in hCG production are dependent on imports of raw material from China.

References

Abbasi-Shavazi, Mohammad Jalal, Marcia C. Inhorn, Hajiieh Bibi Razeghi-Nasrabad, and Ghasem Toloo. 2008. "The 'Iranian ART Revolution': Infertility, Assisted Reproductive Technology, and Third-Party Donation in the Islamic Republic of Iran." *Journal of Middle East Women's Studies* 4 (2): 1–28. https://doi.org/10.2979/MEW.2008.4.2.1.

Abraham, Itty. 2000. "Landscape and Postcolonial Science." *Contributions to Indian Sociology* 34 (2): 163–87. https://doi.org/10.1177%2F006996670003400201.

Abraham, Itty. 2006. "The Contradictory Spaces of Postcolonial Techno-Science." *Economic and Political Weekly* 41 (3): 210–17. https://www.epw.in/journal/2006/03/review-science-policy-review-issues-specials/contradictory-spaces-postcolonial.

Abrahamsson, Sebastian, Filippo Bertoni, Annemarie Mol, and Rebeca Ibáñez Martín. 2015. "Living with Omega-3: New Materialism and Enduring Concerns." *Environment and Planning D: Society and Space* 33 (1): 4–19. https://doi.org/10.1068%2Fd14086p.

Abram, Simone, and Gisa Weszkalnys. 2011. "Introduction: Elusive Promises—Planning in the Contemporary World." *Focaal—Journal of Global and Historical Anthropology* 61:3–18. https://doi.org/10.3167/fcl.2011.610101.

Almeling, Rene. 2007. "Selling Genes, Selling Gender: Egg Agencies, Sperm Banks, and the Medical Market in Genetic Material." *American Sociological Review* 72 (3): 319–40. https://doi.org/10.1177%2F000312240707200301.

Almeling, Rene. 2011. *Sex Cells: The Medical Market for Eggs and Sperm*. Berkeley: University of California Press.

Alter, Joseph S. 1992. *The Wrestler's Body: Identity and Ideology in North India*. Berkeley: University of California Press.

Alter, Joseph S. 2004. *Yoga in Modern India: The Body between Science and Philosophy*. Princeton, NJ: Princeton University Press.

Amrita Bazar Patrika. 1978a. "Test Tube Baby Probe Ordered." October 7, 1978.

Amrita Bazar Patrika. 1978b. "Test Tube Baby Doing Well." October 8, 1978.

Amrita Bazar Patrika. 1978c. "Test Tube Baby: Docs to Explain." October 10, 1978.

Amrita Bazar Patrika. 1978d. "Test Tube Baby." October 11, 1978.

Amrita Bazar Patrika. 1978e. "Mother Not to Undergo Medical Check-Up." November 20, 1978.

Amrita Bazar Patrika. 1978f. "Expert Body Sittings on Test Tube Baby." November 22, 1978.

Amrita Bazar Patrika. 1978g. "Test Tube Baby." December 4, 1978.

Amrita Bazar Patrika. 1978h. "Expert Body Dismisses Claim." December 7, 1978.

Anagnost, Ann S. 2006. "Strange Circulations: The Blood Economy in Rural China." *Economy and Society* 35 (4): 509–29. https://doi.org/10.1080/03085140600960781.

Anand Kumar, T. C. 1997a. "Architect of India's First Test Tube Baby: Dr. Subhas Mukerji (16 January 1931 to 19 July 1981)." *Current Science* 72 (7): 526–31.

Anand Kumar, T. C. 1997b. "The Triumph and Tragedy of Professor Subhas Mukerjee: Professor Subhas Mukerjee Memorial Oration." Delivered at the Third National Congress on Assisted Reproductive Technology and Advances in Infertility, Calcutta, February 8, 1997.

Anand Kumar, T. C. 2004. "In Vitro Fertilization in India." *Current Science* 86 (2): 254–56. https://www.jstor.org/stable/24107860.

Anand Kumar, T. C., C. P. Puri, K. Gopalkrishnan, and I. N. Hinduja. 1988. Letters to the editors. *Journal of In Vitro Fertilization and Embryo Transfer* 5 (6): 376–77.

Anderson, Warwick. 2002. "Introduction: Postcolonial Technoscience." *Social Studies of Science* 32 (5–6): 643–58. https://doi.org/10.1177%2F030631270203200502.

Appadurai, Arjun, ed. 1986. *The Social Life of Things: Commodities in Cultural Perspective.* New York: Cambridge University Press.

Appadurai, Arjun. 1996. *Modernity at Large: Cultural Dimensions of Globalization.* Minneapolis: University of Minnesota Press.

Arnold, David. 1993. *Colonizing the Body: State Medicine and Epidemic Disease in Nineteenth Century India.* Delhi: Oxford University Press.

Arnold, David. 2013. "Nehruvian Science and Postcolonial India." *Isis* 104 (2): 360–70. https://doi.org/10.1086/670954.

Babb, Lawrence A. 1983. "Destiny and Responsibility: Karma in Popular Hinduism." In *Karma: An Anthropological Inquiry*, edited by Charles F. Keyes and E. Valentine Daniel, 163–84. Berkeley: University of California Press.

Bakshi, Ajay, and Lawton R. Burns. 2014. "The Medical Profession in India." In *India's Healthcare Industry: Innovation in Delivery, Financing, and Manufacturing*, edited by Lawton R. Burns, 141–68. Cambridge: Cambridge University Press. https://doi.org/10.1017/cbo9781107360242.005.

Banerjee, Amrita. 2014. "Race and a Transnational Reproductive Caste System: Indian Transnational Surrogacy." *Hypatia* 29 (1): 113–28. https://doi:10.1111/hypa.12056.

Banerjee, Dwaipayan. 2011. "No Biosociality in India." Book review. *BioSocieties* 6 (4): 488–92. https://www.academia.edu/855003/No_Biosociality_in_India.

Banerjee, Sneha. 2015. "Making Feminist Sense of the Commercial Surrogacy 'Industry' in India." PhD thesis, Jawaharlal Nehru University.

Banerjee, Sneha, and Prabha Kotiswaran. 2021. "Divine Labours, Devalued Work: The Continuing Saga of India's Surrogacy Regulation." *Indian Law Review* 5 (1): 85–105. https://doi.org/10.1080/24730580.2020.1843317.

Barad, Karen. 1998. "Getting Real: Technoscientific Practices and the Materialization of Reality." *Differences: A Journal of Feminist Cultural Studies* 10 (2): 87–128. http://www.open.ac.uk/researchprojects/iccm/library/39.html.

Bärnreuther, Sandra. 2016. "Innovations 'Out of Place': Controversies over IVF Beginnings in India between 1978 and 2005." *Medical Anthropology* 35 (1): 73–89. https://doi.org/10.1080/01459740.2015.1094066.

Bärnreuther, Sandra. 2018. "Suitable Substances: How Biobanks (Re)Store Biologicals." *New Genetics and Society* 37 (4): 319–37. https://doi.org/10.1080/14636778.2018.1546572.

Bärnreuther, Sandra. 2019. "When Time Stretches: Waiting and In Vitro Fertilization in India," with photographs by Chhandak Pradhan. *Collection Puruṣārtha* 36:269–85. http://editions.ehess.fr/ouvrages/ouvrage/lhopital-en-asie-du-sud/.

Bärnreuther, Sandra. 2020. "Traders of Gametes, Brokers of Values: Mediating Commercial Gamete Donations in Delhi." *Economy & Society* 49 (3): 455–73. https://doi.org/10.1080/03085147.2020.1743074.

Barrett, Ronald L. 2008. *Aghor Medicine: Pollution, Death, and Healing in Northern India.* Berkeley: University of California Press.

Baru, Rama V. 2000. "Privatisation and Corporatisation." In *Unhealthy Trends: A Symposium on the State of Our Public Health System.* http://www.india-seminar.com/2000/489/489%20baru.htm.

Baru, Rama V. 2001. "Health Sector Reform and Structural Adjustment: A State-Level Analysis." In *Public Health and the Poverty of Reforms: The South Asian Predicament,* edited by Imrana Qadeer, Kasturi Sen, and K. R. Nayar, 211–34. New Delhi: Sage Publications.

Baru, Rama V. 2003. "Privatisation of Health Services: A South Asian Perspective." *Economic and Political Weekly* 38 (42): 4433–37. https://www.jstor.org/stable/4414156?seq=1#metadata_info_tab_contents.

Baru, Rama V. 2006. *Privatisation of Health Care in India: A Comparative Analysis of Orissa, Karnataka and Maharashtra States.* New Delhi: Indian Institute of Public Administration.

Becker, Gay. 1994. "Metaphors in Disrupted Lives: Infertility and Cultural Constructions of Continuity." *Medical Anthropology Quarterly* 8 (4): 383–410. https://www.jstor.org/stable/649087?seq=1#metadata_info_tab_contents.

Becker, Gay. 2000. *The Elusive Embryo: How Women and Men Approach New Reproductive Technologies.* Berkeley: University of California Press.

Bennett, Lynn. 1983. *Dangerous Wives and Sacred Sisters: Social and Symbolic Roles of High-Caste Women in Nepal.* New York: Columbia University Press.

Bergmann, Sven. 2014. *Ausweichrouten der Reproduktion. Biomedizinische Mobilität und die Praxis der Eizellspende.* Berlin: Springer.

Bettendorf, Gerhard, ed. 1995. *Zur Geschichte der Endokrinologie und Reproduktionsmedizin: 256 Biographien und Berichte.* Berlin: Springer.

Bharadwaj, Aditya. 2000. "How Some Indian Baby Makers Are Made: Media Narratives and Assisted Conception in India." *Anthropology and Medicine* 7 (1): 63–78. https://doi.org/10.1080/136484700109359.

Bharadwaj, Aditya. 2002. "Conception Politics: Medical Egos, Media Spotlights, and the Contest over Testtube Firsts in India." In *Infertility around the Globe: New Thinking on Childlessness, Gender, and Reproductive Technologies,* edited by Marcia C. Inhorn and Frank van Balen, 315–34. Berkeley: University of California Press.

Bharadwaj, Aditya. 2003. "Why Adoption Is Not an Option in India: The Visibility of Infertility, the Secrecy of Donor Insemination, and Other Cultural Complexities." *Social Science and Medicine* 56 (9): 1867–80. https://doi.org/10.1016/S0277-9536(02)00210-1.

Bharadwaj, Aditya. 2006. "Sacred Conceptions: Clinical Theodicies, Uncertain Science, and Technologies of Procreation in India." *Culture, Medicine and Psychiatry* 30:451–65. https://doi.org/10.1007/s11013-006-9032-0.

Bharadwaj, Aditya. 2014. "Experimental Subjectification: The Pursuit of Human Embryonic Stem Cells in India." *Ethnos* 79 (1): 84–107. https://doi.org/10.1080/00141844.2013.806947.

Bharadwaj, Aditya. 2016. *Conceptions: Infertility and Procreative Technologies in India.* New York: Berghahn Books.

Bharadwaj, Aditya, and Peter E. Glasner. 2009. *Local Cells, Global Science: The Rise of Embryonic Stem Cell Research in India.* London: Routledge.

Birenbaum-Carmeli, Daphna, and Marcia C. Inhorn. 2009. *Assisting Reproduction, Testing Genes: Global Encounters with New Biotechnologies.* Oxford: Berghahn Books.

Bloch, Maurice. 2008. "Truth and Sight: Generalizing without Universalizing." *Journal of the Royal Anthropological Institute* 14 (S1): S22–S32. https://doi.org/10.1111/j.1467-9655.2008.00490.x.

Böck, Monika, and Aparna Rao. 2000. "Indigenous Models and Kinship Theories: An Introduction to a South Asian Perspective." In *Culture, Creation and Procreation: Concepts of Kinship in South Asian Practice,* edited by Monika Böck and Aparna Rao, 1–52. New York: Berghahn Books.

Boiso, Irene, Anna Vega, and Robert G. Edwards. 2002. "Fundamentals of Human Embryonic Growth In Vitro and the Selection of High-Quality Embryos for

Transfer." Reproductive BioMedicine Online 5 (3): 328–50. https://www.rbmojour nal.com/article/S1472-6483(10)61841-X/pdf.

Bonhomme, Julien. 2012. "The Dangers of Anonymity: Witchcraft, Rumor, and Modernity in Africa." *HAU: Journal of Ethnographic Theory* 2 (2): 205–33. https://doi.org/10.14318/hau2.2.012.

Burghardt, Scout, and Kerstin Tote. 2010. "Zwischen Risikovermeidung, Normalisierung und Markt: Spenderauswahl und *matching* in Samenbanken." In *Samenbanken—Samenspender: Ethnographische und Historische Perspektiven auf Männlichkeiten in der Reproduktionsmedizin*, edited by Michi Knecht, Scout Burghardt, Anna Frederike Heinitz, and Sebastian Mohr, 142–62. Münster: LIT Verlag.

Burns, Lawton R. 2014. "India's Healthcare Industry: An Overview of the Value Chain." In *India's Healthcare Industry: Innovation in Delivery, Financing, and Manufacturing*, edited by Lawton R. Burns, 59–138. Cambridge: Cambridge University Press.

Burns, Lawton R., Bhuvan Srinivasan, and Mandar Vaidya. 2014. "India's Hospital Sector: The Journey from Public to Private Healthcare Delivery." In *India's Healthcare Industry: Innovation in Delivery, Financing, and Manufacturing*, edited by Lawton R. Burns, 169–218. Cambridge: Cambridge University Press.

Carsten, Janet. 2001. "Substantivism, Antisubstantivism, and Anti-Antisubstantivism." In *Relative Values: Reconfiguring Kinship Studies*, edited by Sarah Franklin and Susan McKinnon, 29–53. Durham, NC: Duke University Press.

Carsten, Janet. 2004. *After Kinship*. Cambridge: Cambridge University Press.

Chakrabarty, Dipesh. 2000. *Provincializing Europe: Postcolonial Thought and Historical Difference*. Princeton, NJ: Princeton University Press.

Chakravarthi, Indira. 2010. "Corporate Presence in the Healthcare Sector in India." *Social Medicine* 5 (4): 192–204. https://www.socialmedicine.info/index.php/ socialmedicine/article/view/502/1030.

Chatterjee, Siddhartha. 2011. "Prof. Robert Edwards, Nobel Laureate in Medicine 2010—Tribute of an Indian with Joy and Sorrow." *Al Ameen Journal of Medical Sciences* 4 (1): 1–2. https://doaj.org/article/5f66fc2482fa4ec5b7d5fb0e802f4126.

Chaudhuri, Sudip. 2005. *The WTO and India's Pharmaceuticals Industry: Patent Protection, TRIPS and Developing Countries*. New Delhi: Oxford University Press.

Chowdhury, I. 2006. "Mukerji, Subhas." In *Dictionary of Medical Biography*, edited by William F. Bynum and Helen Bynum. Westport, CT: Greenwood.

Churchill Archives Centre. n.d. Papers of Robert Edwards, EDWS 2/4/1.

Clarke, Adele. 1998. *Disciplining Reproduction: Modernity, American Life Sciences and the Problems of Sex*. Berkeley: University of California Press.

Clarke, Morgan. 2008. "New Kinship, Islam and the Liberal Tradition: Sexual Morality and New Reproductive Technology in Lebanon." *Journal of the Royal Anthropological Institute* 14 (1): 153–69. https://doi.org/10.1111/j.1467-9655.2007.00483.x.

Clarke, Morgan. 2009. *Islam and New Kinship: Reproductive Technology and the Shariah in Lebanon*. New York: Berghahn Books.

Cohen, Lawrence. 1994. "Whodunit?—Violence and the Myth of Fingerprints: Comment on Harding." *Configurations* 2 (2): 343–47. https://doi.org/10.1353/con.1994.0022.

Cohen, Lawrence. 2005. "Operability, Bioavailibility, and Exception." In *Global Assemblages: Technology, Politics, and Ethics as Anthropological Problems*, edited by Aihwa Ong and Stephen J. Collier, 79–90. Malden, MA: Blackwell.

Colen, Shellee. 1995. "'Like a Mother to Them': Stratified Reproduction and West Indian Childcare Workers and Employers in New York." In *Conceiving the New World Order: The Global Politics of Reproduction*, edited by Faye Ginsburg and Rayna Rapp, 78–102. Berkeley: University of California Press.

Comaroff, Jean, and John L. Comaroff. 1999. "Occult Economies and the Violence of Abstraction: Notes from the South African Postcolony." *American Ethnologist* 26 (2): 279–303. https://doi.org/10.1525/ae.1999.26.2.279.

Comaroff, Jean, and John L. Comaroff. 2012. "Theory from the South: A Rejoinder." *Cultural Anthropology Online*, February 25, 2012. https://culanth.org/fieldsights/theory-from-the-south-a-rejoinder.

Connor, Linda H. 2001. "Healing Powers in Contemporary Asia." In *Healing Powers and Modernity: Traditional Medicine, Shamanism and Science in Asian Societies*, edited by Linda H. Connor and Geoffrey Samuel, 1–21. London: Bergin & Garvey.

Cooper, Melinda E. 2008. *Life as Surplus: Biotechnology and Capitalism in the Neoliberal Era*. Seattle: University of Washington Press.

Cooper, Melinda, and Catherine Waldby. 2014. *Clinical Labor: Tissue Donors and Research Subjects in the Global Bioeconomy*. Durham, NC: Duke University Press.

Copeman, Jacob. 2013. "South Asian Tissue Economies." *Contemporary South Asia* 21 (3): 195–213. https://doi.org/10.1080/09584935.2013.826628.

Copeman, Jacob, and Dwaipayan Banerjee. 2019. Hematologies: The Political Life of Blood in India. Ithaca, NY: Cornell University Press.

Cresswell, Tim. 2015. *Place: An Introduction*. 2nd ed. Chichester: Wiley Blackwell.

Cromer, Risa. 2018. "Saving Embryos in Stem Cell Science and Embryo Adoption." *New Genetics and Society* 37 (4): 362–86. https://doi.org/10.1080/14636778.2018.1546574.

Cross, Jamie. 2014. *Dream Zones: Anticipating Capitalism and Development in India*. London: Pluto.

Daniel, E. Valentine. 1984. *Fluid Signs: Being a Person the Tamil Way*. Berkeley: University of California Press.

Das, Veena. 1995. "National Honor and Practical Kinship: Unwanted Women and Children." In *Conceiving the New World Order: The Global Politics of Reproduction*, edited by Faye Ginsburg and Rayna Rapp, 212–33. Berkeley: University of California Press.

Das, Veena. 2012. "Ordinary Ethics." In *A Companion to Moral Anthropology*, edited by Didier Fassin, 133–49. Chichester: Wiley-Blackwell.

Daston, Lorraine J., and Peter Galison. 2010. *Objectivity*. Cambridge: Zone Books.

Datta, D. 2010. "Infertility on the Rise." *India Today International*, July 5, 2010.

Deccan Herald. 2014. "Film Documents Life of India's First Test-Tube Baby Creator." November 14, 2014.

de Lacey, Sheryl. 2002. "IVF as Lottery or Investment: Contesting Metaphors in Discourses of Infertility." *Nursing Inquiry* 9 (1): 43–51. https://doi.org/10.1046/j.1440-1800.2002.00126.x.

Deomampo, Daisy. 2016. *Transnational Reproduction: Race, Kinship and Commercial Surrogacy in India*. New York: NYU Press.

Douglas, Mary. (1966) 2002. *Purity and Danger: An Analysis of the Concepts of Pollution and Taboo*. London: Routledge.

Dube, Leela. 1988. "On the Construction of Gender: Hindu Girls in Patrilineal India." *Economic and Political Weekly* 23 (18): WS11–WS19. https://www.epw.in/journal/1988/18/review-womens-studies-review-issues/construction-gender.html.

Eckert, Julia. 2012. "Rumours of Rights." In *Law against the State: Ethnographic Forays into Law's Transformations*, edited by Julia Eckert, Brian Donahoe, Christian Strümpell, and Zerrin Özlem Biner, 147–70. Cambridge: Cambridge University Press.

Edwards, Jeanette. 2000. *Born and Bred: Idioms of Kinship and New Reproductive Technologies in England*. Oxford: Oxford University Press.

Edwards, Jeanette. 2014. "Undoing Kinship." In *Relatedness in Assisted Reproduction: Families, Origins and Identities*, edited by Tabitha Freeman, Susanna Graham, Fatemeh Ebtehaj, and Martin Richards, 44–60. Cambridge: Cambridge University Press.

Edwards, Robert G. 2001. "The Bumpy Road to Human In Vitro Fertilization." *Nature Medicine* 7 (10): 1091–94. https://doi.org/10.1038/nm1001-1091.

Emirbayer, Mustafa. 1997. "Manifesto for a Relational Sociology." *American Journal of Sociology* 103 (2): 281–317. https://www.jstor.org/stable/10.1086/231209?seq=1 #metadata_info_tab_contents.

Ernst and Young LLP. 2015. "Call for Action: Expanding IVF Treatment in India." July.

Fassin, Didier. 2009. "Another Politics of Life Is Possible." *Theory, Culture and Society* 26 (5): 44–60. https://doi.org/10.1177%2F0263276409106349.

Foucault, Michel. 1973. *The Birth of the Clinic: An Archaeology of Medical Perception*. New York: Random House.

Franklin, Sarah. 1997. *Embodied Progress: A Cultural Account of Assisted Conception*. London: Routledge.

Franklin, Sarah. 2006. "The Cyborg Embryo: Our Path to Transbiology." *Theory, Culture and Society* 23 (7–8): 167–87. https://doi.org/10.1177%2F0263276406069230.

Franklin, Sarah. 2013. *Biological Relatives: IVF, Stem Cells, and the Future of Kinship*. Durham, NC: Duke University Press.

Franklin, Sarah, and Marcia C. Inhorn. 2016. "Symposium: IVF—Global Histories; Introduction." *Reproductive BioMedicine and Society Online* 2:1–7. https://doi.org/10.1016/j.rbms.2016.05.001.

Franklin, Sarah, and Susan McKinnon, eds. 2001. *Relative Values: Reconfiguring Kinship Studies*. Durham, NC: Duke University Press.

Franklin, Sarah, and Helena Ragoné, eds. 1998. *Reproducing Reproduction: Kinship, Power, and Technological Innovation*. Philadelphia: University of Pennsylvania Press.

Franklin, Sarah, and Celia Roberts. 2006. *Born and Made: An Ethnography of Preimplantation Genetic Diagnosis*. Princeton, NJ: Princeton University Press.

Gaudillière, Jean-Paul. 2004. "Genesis and Development of a Biomedical Object: Styles of Thought, Styles of Work and the History of the Sex Steroids." *Studies in History and Philosophy of Biological & Biomedical Sciences* 35:525–43. https://doi.org/10.1016/j.shpsc.2004.06.003.

Gaudillière, Jean-Paul. 2005. "Better Prepared Than Synthesized: Adolf Butenandt, Schering Ag and the Transformation of Sex Steroids into Drugs (1930–1946)." *Studies in History and Philosophy of Biological & Biomedical Sciences* 36:612–44. https://doi.org/10.1016/j.shpsc.2005.09.006.

Ginsburg, Faye D., and Rayna Rapp. 1995. *Conceiving the New World Order: The Global Politics of Reproduction*. Berkeley: University of California Press.

Gleicher, Norbert, Mary Vietzke, and Andrea Vidali. 2003. "Bye-Bye Urinary Gonadotrophins? Recombinant FSH: A Real Progress in Ovulation Induction and IVF?" *Human Reproduction* 18 (3): 476–82. https://doi.org/10.1093/humrep/deg099.

Gooptu, Nandini. 2013. *Enterprise Culture in Neoliberal India: Studies in Youth, Class, Work and Media*. London: Routledge.

Gosh, A. 2005. "It's Official: Kanupriya's India's First Test-Tube Girl." *DNA*, August 19, 2005.

Government of India. 2003. *Science and Technology Policy 2003*. New Delhi.

Government of India. 2005. *National Guidelines for Accreditation, Supervision & Regulation of ART Clinics in India*. New Delhi.

Government of India. 2010. "PM Inaugurates 97th Indian Science Congress." Press release, January 3, 2010. http://pib.nic.in/newsite/erelease.aspx?relid=56577.

Government of India. 2020. Assisted Reproductive Technologies (Regulation) Bill, 2020. New Delhi.

Gupta, Jyotsna A. 2011. "Exploring Appropriation of 'Surplus' Ova and Embryos in Indian IVF Clinics." *New Genetics and Society* 30 (2): 167–80. https://doi.org/10.1080/14636778.2011.574373.

Gusterson, Hugh. 1997. "Studying Up Revisited." *PoLAR: Political and Legal Anthropology Review* 20 (1): 114–19. https://doi.org/10.1525/pol.1997.20.1.114.

Hacking, Ian. 1981. "Do We See through a Microscope?" Pacific Philosophical Quarterly 63:305–22. https://doi.org/10.1111/j.1468-0114.1981.tb00070.x.

Hampshire, Kate, and Bob Simpson. 2015. *Assisted Reproductive Technologies in the Third Phase: Global Encounters and Emerging Moral Worlds*. New York: Berghahn Books.

Handwerker, Lisa. 2002. "The Politics of Making Modern Babies in China: Reproductive Technologies and the 'New' Eugenics." In *Infertility around the Globe*, edited by Marcia C. Inhorn and Frank van Balen, 298–314. Berkeley: University of California Press.

Haraway, Donna J. 1994. "A Game of Cat's Cradle: Science Studies, Feminist Theory, Cultural Studies." *Configurations* 2 (1): 59–71. https://doi.org/10.1353/con.1994.0009.

Haraway, Donna. 2012. "Awash in Urine: DES and Premarin® in Multispecies Response-Ability." *Women's Studies Quarterly* 40 (1&2): 301–16. https://doi.org/10.1353/wsq.2012.0005.

Hayden, Cori. 2013. "Distinctively Similar: A Generic Problem." *UC Davis Law Journal* 44 (2): 601–32. https://lawreview.law.ucdavis.edu/issues/47/2/Symposium/47-2_Hayden.pdf.

Heimerl, Birgit. 2013. *Die Ultraschallsprechstunde: Eine Ethnografie pränataldiagnostischer Situationen*. Bielefeld: Transcript.

Hess, Linda. 1988. "The Poet, the People, and the Western Scholar: Influence of a Sacred Drama and Text on Social Values in North India." *Theatre Journal* 40 (2): 236–53. https://doi.org/10.2307/3207659.

The Hindu. 2011. "Bourn Hall Clinic Opens First IVF Centre in India." April 14, 2011.

Hodges, Sarah. 2013a. "Umbilical Cord Blood Banking and Its Interruptions: Notes from Chennai, India." *Economy and Society* 42 (4): 651–70. https://doi.org/10.1080/03085147.2013.772759.

Hodges, Sarah. 2013b. "'It All Changed after Apollo': Healthcare Myths and Their Making in Contemporary India." *Indian Journal of Medical Ethics* 10 (4): 242–49. https://doi.org/10.20529/ijme.2013.073.

Hopkins, Terence K., and Immanuel Wallerstein. 1986. "Commodity Chains in the World-Economy Prior to 1800." Review (Fernand Braudel Center) 10 (1): 157–70. https://www.jstor.org/stable/40241052.

Indian Council of Medical Research. 2000. "Need and Feasibility of Providing Assisted Technologies for Infertility Management in Resource-Poor Settings." *ICMR Bulletin* 30 (6–7). https://main.icmr.nic.in/sites/default/files/icmr_bulletins/bujunjuly00.pdf.

Inhorn, Marcia C. 1994. *Quest for Conception: Gender, Infertility, and Egyptian Medical Traditions*. Philadelphia: University of Pennsylvania Press.

Inhorn, Marcia C. 1996. *Infertility and Patriarchy: The Cultural Politics of Gender and Family Life in Egypt*. Philadelphia: University of Pennsylvania Press.

Inhorn, Marcia C. 2003a. "Global Infertility and the Globalization of New Reproductive Technologies: Illustrations from Egypt." *Social Science and Medicine* 56 (9): 1837–51. https://doi.org/10.1016/S0277-9536(02)00208-3.

Inhorn, Marcia C. 2003b. *Local Babies, Global Science. Gender, Religion, and In Vitro Fertilization in Egypt*. New York: Routledge.

Inhorn, Marcia C. 2004. "Privacy, Privatization, and the Politics of Patronage: Ethnographic Challenges to Penetrating the Secret World of Middle Eastern, Hospital-
Based In Vitro Fertilization." *Social Science and Medicine* 59 (10): 2095–108.
https://doi.org/10.1016/j.socscimed.2004.03.012.

Inhorn, Marcia C. 2006. "Making Muslim Babies: IVF and Gamete Donation in Sunni
versus Shia Islam." *Culture, Medicine and Psychiatry* 30 (4): 427–50. https://
dx.doi.org/10.1007%2Fs11013-006-9027-x.

Inhorn, Marcia C. 2007. *Reproductive Disruptions: Gender, Technology, and Biopolitics
in the New Millennium.* New York: Berghahn Books.

Inhorn, Marcia C. 2012. *The New Arab Man: Emergent Masculinities, Technologies, and
Islam in the Middle East.* Princeton, NJ: Princeton University Press.

Inhorn, Marcia C. 2015. *Cosmopolitan Conceptions: IVF Sojourns in Global Dubai.*
Durham, NC: Duke University Press.

Inhorn, Marcia C., and Frank van Balen. 2002. *Infertility around the Globe: New Thinking on Childlessness, Gender, and Reproductive Technologies.* Berkeley: University
of California Press.

Inhorn, Marcia C., and Daphna Birenbaum-Carmeli. 2008. "Assisted Reproductive
Technologies and Culture Change." *Annual Review of Anthropology* 37:177–96.
https://doi.org/10.1146/annurev.anthro.37.081407.085230.

Inscape. 2007. "40 Years Together." Special edition, August 2007. Organon India.

International Federation of Fertility Societies. 2019. "International Federation of Fertility Societies' Surveillance (IFFS) 2019: Global Trends in Reproductive Policy
and Practice, 8th Edition." *Global Reproductive Health* 4 (1): Supplement Article.
https://doi.org/10.1097/GRH.0000000000000029.

Jain, Madhu. 1986. "First Made-in-India Test-Tube Baby to Be Born Next Month in
Bombay." *India Today*, July 15, 1986.

Joseph, Reji K., and K. V. K. Ranganathan. 2016. *Trends in Foreign Investment in
Healthcare Sector of India.* Working Paper 187. New Delhi: Institute for Studies
in Industrial Development. http://111.93.232.162/pdf/WP187.pdf.

Kahn, Susan Martha. 2000. *Reproducing Jews: A Cultural Account of Assisted Conception in Israel.* Durham, NC: Duke University Press.

Kaspar, Heidi, and Sunita Reddy. 2017. "Spaces of Connectivity: The Formation of
Medical Travel Destinations in Delhi National Capital Region (India)." *Asian
Pacific Viewpoint* 58 (2): 228–41. https://doi.org/10.1111/apv.12159.

Kleinman, Arthur. 1999. "Moral Experience and Ethical Reflection: Can Ethnography
Reconcile Them? A Quandary for 'the New Bioethics.'" *Dædalus* 128 (4): 69–97.
https://www.jstor.org/stable/20027589.

Klotz, Maren. 2014. *(K)information: Gamete Donation and Kinship Knowledge in Germany and Britain.* Frankfurt: Campus Verlag.

Knecht, Michi, Maren Klotz, and Stefan Beck. 2012. *Reproductive Technologies as
Global Form: Ethnographies of Knowledge, Practices, and Transnational Encounters.* Frankfurt: Campus Verlag.

Kohler, Robert E. 2002. *Landscapes and Labscapes: Exploring the Lab-Field Border in
Biology.* Chicago: University of Chicago Press.

Konrad, Monica. 2005. *Nameless Relations: Anonymity, Melanesia and Reproductive Gift
Exchange between British Ova Donors and Recipients.* New York: Berghahn Books.

Kroløkke, Charlotte. 2018. *Global Fluids: The Cultural Politics of Reproductive Waste
and Value.* New York: Berghahn Books.

Kumar, Anil. 2001. "The Indian Drug Industry under the Raj, 1860–1920." In *Health,
Medicine and Empire: Perspectives on Colonial Empire*, edited by Biswamoy Pati
and Mark Harrison, 356–85. Hyderabad: Orient Longman.

Kuriyama, Shigehisa. 1999. *The Expressiveness of the Body, and the Divergence of Greek and Chinese Medicine*. New York: Zone Books.

Lamb, Sarah. 1997. "The Making and Unmaking of Persons: Notes on Aging and Gender in North India." *Ethos* 25 (3): 279–302. https://doi.org/10.1525/eth.1997.25.3.279.

Lambek, Michael. 1997. "Knowledge and Practice in Mayotte: An Overview." *Cultural Dynamics* 9 (2): 131–48. https://doi.org/10.1177%2F092137409700900201.

Lambek, Michael. 2010. *Ordinary Ethics: Anthropology, Language, and Action*. New York: Fordham University Press.

Lambert, Helen. 2000. "Sentiment and Substance in North Indian Forms of Relatedness." In *Cultures of Relatedness: New Approaches to the Study of Kinship*, edited by Janet Carsten, 73–89. Cambridge: Cambridge University Press.

Laqueur, Thomas W. 2000. "'From Generation to Generation': Imagining Connectedness in the Age of Reproductive Technologies." In *Biotechnology and Culture: Bodies, Anxieties, Ethics*, edited by Paul Brodwin, 75–98. Bloomington: Indiana University Press.

Latour, Bruno. 1983. "Give Me a Laboratory and I Will Raise the World." In *Science Observed: Perspectives on the Social Study of Science*, edited by Karin D. Knorr Cetina and Michael J. Mulkay, 141–70. Beverly Hills, CA: Sage Publications.

Latour, Bruno. 1986. "Visualisation and Cognition: Drawing Things Together." In *Knowledge and Society: Studies in the Sociology of Culture Past and Present*, edited by Henrika Kuklick. Greenwich, CT: Jai Press.

Latour, Bruno. 1987. *Science in Action: How to Follow Scientists and Engineers through Society*. Cambridge, MA: Harvard University Press.

Latour, Bruno. 1993. *We Have Never Been Modern*. New York: Harvester Wheatsheaf.

Latour, Bruno. 1999. *Pandora's Hope: Essays on the Reality of Science Studies*. Cambridge, MA: Harvard University Press.

Latour, Bruno, and Steve Woolgar. 1986. *Laboratory Life: The Construction of Scientific Facts*. Princeton, NJ: Princeton University Press.

Laveaga, Gabriela Soto. 2005. "Uncommon Trajectories: Steroid Hormones, Mexican Peasants, and the Search for a Wild Yam." *Studies in History and Philosophy of Biological & Biomedical Sciences* 36:743–60. https://doi.org/10.1016/j.shpsc.2005.09.007.

Law, John, and Annemarie Mol. 2001. "Situating Technoscience: An Inquiry into Spatialities." *Environment and Planning D: Society and Space* 19 (5): 609–21. https://doi.org/10.1068%2Fd243t.

Leão, Rogério de Barros Ferreira, and Sandro C. Esteves. 2015. "Gonadotropin in Assisted Reproduction: An Evolution Perspective." In *Unexplained Infertility*, edited by Glenn L. Schattman, Sandro C. Esteves, and Ashok Agarwal, 293–322. Berlin: Springer.

Lefebvre, Bertrand. 2008. "The Indian Corporate Hospitals: Touching Middle Class Lives." In *Patterns of Middle Class Consumption in India and China*, edited by Christophe Jaffrelot and Peter van der Veer, 88–109. New Delhi: Sage Publications.

Lefebvre, Bertrand. 2010. "Hospital Chains in India: The Coming of Age?" *Asie Visions* 23. Working paper. https://www.ifri.org/en/publications/enotes/asie-visions/hospital-chains-india-coming-age.

Lindemann, Gesa. 2002. *Die Grenzen des Sozialen: Zur sozio-technischen Konstruktion von Leben und Tod in der Intensivmedizin*. Munich: Wilhelm Fink Verlag.

Livingstone, David N. 2003. *Putting Science in Its Place: Geographies of Scientific Knowledge*. Chicago: University of Chicago Press.

Livingstone, Julie. 2012. *Improvising Medicine: An African Oncology Ward in an Emerging Cancer Epidemic*. Durham, NC: Duke University Press.

Livneh, Neri. 2002. "The Good Father." *Haaretz*, May 30, 2002. https://www.haaretz.com/1.5181405.

Lunenfeld, Bruno. 2009. "60 Years of Gonadotrophins." *Focus on Reproduction*, May 2009.

Lunenfeld, Bruno. 2013. "Management of Infertility: Past, Present and Future (from a Personal Perspective)." *Reproductive Medicine and Endocrinology* 10 (1): 13–22. https://www.semanticscholar.org/paper/Management-of-Infertility%3A-Past%2C-Present-and-Future-Lunenfeld/6b50325fc186c0e9f8d4e3e0cdb9677e082145de.

Majumdar, Anindita. 2017. *Transnational Commercial Surrogacy and the (Un)Making of Kin in India*. Delhi: Oxford University Press.

Mamo, Laura. 2005. "Biomedicalizing Kinship: Sperm Banks and the Creation of Affinity-Ties." *Science as Culture* 14 (3): 237–64. https://doi.org/10.1080/09505430500216833.

Marcus, George E. 1995. "Ethnography in/of the World System: The Emergence of Multi-Sited Ethnography." *Annual Review of Anthropology* 24:95–117. https://www.jstor.org/stable/2155931.

Marriott, McKim. 1968. "Caste Ranking and Food Transactions: A Matrix Analysis." In *Structure and Change in Indian Society*, edited by Milton B. Singer and Bernard S. Cohn, 133–72. New York: Wenner-Gren Foundation for Anthropological Research.

Marriott, McKim. 1976. "Hindu Transactions: Diversity without Dualism." In *Transaction and Meaning: Directions in the Anthropology of Exchange and Symbolic Behavior*, edited by Bruce Kapferer, 109–42. Philadelphia: Institute for the Study of Human Issues.

Marriott, McKim. 1990. "Constructing an Indian Ethnosociology." In *India through Hindu Categories*, edited by McKim Marriott, 1–40. New Delhi: Sage Publications.

Marriott, McKim, and Ronald Inden. 1977. "Toward an Ethnosociology of South Asian Caste Systems." In *The New Wind: Changing Identities in South Asia*, edited by Kenneth David, 227–38. The Hague: Mouton.

Marsland, Rebecca, and Ruth Prince. 2012. "What Is Life Worth? Exploring Biomedical Interventions, Survival, and the Politics of Life." *Medical Anthropology Quarterly* 26 (4): 453–69. https://doi.org/10.1111/maq.12001.

Martin, Emily. 1987. *The Woman in the Body: A Cultural Analysis of Reproduction*. Boston: Beacon.

Martin, Emily. 1998. "Anthropology and the Cultural Study of Science." *Science, Technology, and Human Values* 23 (1): 24–44. https://doi.org/10.1177%2F016224399802300102.

Marx, Karl. (1867) 1990. *Capital: A Critique of Political Economy*. Vol. 1. London: Penguin Books.

Mascarenhas, Maya, Seth Flaxman, Ties Boerma, Sheryl Vanderpoel, and Gretchen Stevens. 2012. "National, Regional, and Global Trends in Infertility Prevalence since 1990: A Systematic Analysis of 277 Health Surveys." *PLOS Medicine* 9 (12): e1001356. https://doi.org/10.1371/journal.pmed.1001356.

Massey, Doreen. 2005. *For Space*. London: Sage Publications.

Mazumdar, Mainak. 2013. *Performance of Pharmaceutical Companies in India: A Critical Analysis of Industrial Structure, Firm Specific Resources, and Emerging Strategies*. Berlin: Springer.

M'charek, Amade. 2013. "Beyond Fact or Fiction: On the Materiality of Race in Practice." *Cultural Anthropology* 28 (3): 420–42. https://doi.org/10.1111/cuan.12012.

McNeil, Maureen. 2005. "Introduction: Postcolonial Technoscience." *Science as Culture* 14 (2): 105–12. https://doi.org/10.1080/09505430500110770.

Merleau-Ponty, Noémie. 2017. "Féconder in vitro dans des laboratoires en Inde et en France. Une somatotechnique?" *Ethnologie Française* 47 (3): 509–18. https://doi.org/10.3917/ethn.173.0509.

Michaels, Axel. 2006. *Der Hinduismus: Geschichte und Gegenwart.* Munich: C. H. Beck.

Miller. Daniel. 2007. "What Is a Relationship? Is Kinship Negotiated Experience?" *Ethnos* 72 (4): 535–54. https://doi.org/10.1080/00141840701768334.

Moeders voor Moeders. n.d.a. Accessed April 4, 2021. Website. https://www.moedersvoor moeders.nl/.

Moeders voor Moeders. n.d.b. "Verhandeling over Gonadatrope Hormonen en de Winning van Pregnyl en Humegon."

Mohr, Sebastian. 2016. "Containing Sperm—Managing Legitimacy: Lust, Disgust, and Hybridity at Danish Sperm Banks." *Journal of Contemporary Ethnography* 45 (3): 319–42. https://doi.org/10.1177%2F0891241614558517.

Mohr, Sebastian. 2018. *Being a Sperm Donor: Masculinity, Sexuality, and Biosociality in Denmark.* New York: Berghahn Books.

Mol, Annemarie. 2008. *The Logic of Care: Health and the Problem of Patient Choice.* London: Routledge.

Moll, Tessa. 2019. "Making a Match: Curating Race in South African Gamete Donation." *Medical Anthropology* 38 (7): 588–602. https://doi.org/10.1080/01459740.2019. 1643853.

Morgan, Lynn M. 2009. *Icons of Life: A Cultural History of Human Embryos.* Berkeley: University of California Press.

Morgan, Lynn M. 2013. "The Potentiality Principle from Aristotle to Abortion." *Current Anthropology* 54 (S7): 15–25. https://doi.org/10.1086/670804.

Morgan, Lynn M., and Elizabeth F. Roberts. 2012. "Reproductive Governance in Latin America." *Anthropology and Medicine* 19 (2): 241–54. https://doi.org/10.1080/13 648470.2012.675046.

Mukherjee, Manjeer, and Sarojini B. Nadimipally. 2006. "Assisted Reproductive Technologies in India." *Development* 49 (4): 128–34. https://doi.org/10.1057/palgrave.devel opment.1100303.

Mukherjee, S., and S. C. Lodh, eds. 2001. *Architect of India's First Test Tube Baby.* Kolkata.

Mukherjee, S., S. Mukherjee, and S. K. Bhattacharya. 1978. "The Feasibility of Long Term Cryogenic Freezing of Viable Human Embryos—a Brief Pilot Study Report." *Indian Journal of Cryogenics* 3 (1): 80.

Mulgaonkar, Veena B. 2001. "Childless Couples in the Slums of Mumbai: An Interdisciplinary Study." *Asia-Pacific Population Journal* 16 (2): 141–60. https://doi.org/10.18356/9b443b45-en.

Murphy, Michelle. 2008. "Chemical Regimes of Living." *Environmental History* 13 (4): 695–703. https://www.jstor.org/stable/25473297.

Nader, Laura. 1972. "Up the Anthropologist—Perspectives Gained from Studying Up." In *Reinventing Anthropology*, edited by Dell Hymes, 284–311. New York: Pantheon Books.

Nagral, Sanjay. 2012. "Doctors in Entrepreneurial Gowns." *Economic and Political Weekly* 47 (36): 10–12. https://www.jstor.org/stable/41720102.

Nanda, Meera. 2016. *Science in Saffron: Skeptical Essays on History of Science.* Gurgaon: Three Essays Collective.

National Archives of India. 1977. "M/s. Organon (India) Ltd., Calcutta—Industrial License for the Manufacture of Steroids Hormones in Bulk of Their Forms." File no. CIL:28/77/LA II; identifier PR_000002841162.

National Institute for Research in Reproductive Health. n.d. "History." Accessed April 4, 2021. http://www.nirrh.res.in/newweb/history/.

Neveling, Patrick. 2014. "Structural Contingencies and Untimely Coincidences in the Making of Neoliberal India: The Kandla Free Trade Zone, 1965–91." *Contributions to Indian Sociology* 48 (1): 17–43. https://doi.org/10.1177%2F0069966713 502420.

Nobel Assembly. 2010. Press release. October 4, 2010. http://www.nobelprize.org/ nobel_prizes/medicine/laureates/2010/press.html.

Nordlund, Christer. 2015. "The Moral Economy of a Miracle Drug: On Exchange Relationships between Medical Science and the Pharmaceutical Industry in the 1940s." In *Value Practices in the Life Sciences and Medicine*, edited by Isabelle Dussauge, Claes-Fredrik Helgesson, and Francis Lee, 49–70. Oxford: Oxford University Press.

Novas, Carlos. 2006. "The Political Economy of Hope: Patients' Organisations, Science and Biovalue." *BioSocieties* 1 (3): 289–305. https://doi.org/10.1017/S174585520 6003024.

Novick, Tamar. 2018. "Die Entdeckung des Urins." In *Nach Feierabend: Zürcher Jahrbuch für Wissensgeschichte 14*, edited by Michael Hagner and Christoph Hoffmann, 139–50. Zürich: Diaphanes.

Ombelet, Willem. 2007. "Affordable IVF for Developing Countries." *Reproductive BioMedicine Online* 15 (3): 257–65. https://doi.org/10.1016/S1472-6483(10)60 337-9.

Ombelet, Willem. 2015. "Global Access to Reproductive Technologies and Infertility Care in Developing Countries." In *Assisted Reproductive Technologies in the Third Phase: Global Encounters and Emerging Moral Worlds*, edited by Kate Hampshire and Bob Simpson, 105–18. New York: Berghahn Books.

Ong, Aihwa, and Stephen J. Collier. 2005. *Global Assemblages: Technology, Politics, and Ethics as Anthropological Problems*. Malden, MA: Blackwell.

Oudshoorn, Nelly. 1994. *Beyond the Natural Body: An Archaeology of Sex Hormones*. New York: Routledge.

Pande, Amrita. 2009. "It May Be Her Eggs but It's My Blood: Surrogates and Everyday Forms of Kinship in India." *Qualitative Sociology* 32 (4): 379–97. https://doi. org/10.1007/s11133-009-9138-0.

Pande, Amrita. 2014. *Wombs in Labor: Transnational Commercial Surrogacy in India*. New York: Columbia University Press.

Parry, Bronwyn. 2018. "Surrogate Labour: Exceptional for Whom?" *Economy and Society* 47 (2): 214–33. https://doi.org/10.1080/03085147.2018.1487180.

Parry, Jonathan P. 1994. *Death in Banaras*. Cambridge: Cambridge University Press.

Pashigian, Melissa J. 2009. "The Womb, Infertility and the Vicissitudes of Kin-Relatedness in Vietnam." *Journal of Vietnamese Studies* 4 (2): 34–68. https://doi.org/10.1525/ vs.2009.4.2.34.

Patel, Tulsi. 1994. *Fertility Behaviour: Population and Society in a Rajasthan Village*. Delhi: Oxford University Press.

Patel, Tulsi. 2007. "Introduction: Gender Relations, NRTs and Female Foeticide in India." In *Sex-Selective Abortion in India: Gender, Society and New Reproductive Technologies*, edited by Tulsi Patel, 27–60. London: Sage Publications.

Petryna, Adriana. 2011. "The Competitive Logic of Global Clinical Trials." *Social Research* 78 (3): 949–74. https://muse.jhu.edu/article/528161.

Porqueres i Gené, Enric, and Jérôme Wilgaux. 2009. "Incest, Embodiment, Genes and Kinship." In *European Kinship in the Age of Biotechnology*, edited by J. Edwards and C. Salazar, 112–27. New York: Berghahn Books.

Practice Committee of the American Society for Reproductive Medicine. 2008. "Gonadotropin Preparations: Past, Present, and Future Perspectives." *Fertility and Sterility* 90 (5) Supplement: S13–S20. https://doi.org/10.1016/j.fertnstert.2008.08.031.

Prakash, Gyan. 1999. *Another Reason: Science and the Imagination of Modern India*. Princeton, NJ: Princeton University Press.

Prasad, Amit. 2005. "Scientific Culture in the 'Other' Theatre of 'Modern Science': An Analysis of the Culture of Magnetic Resonance Imaging Research in India." *Social Studies of Science* 3 (3): 463–89. https://doi.org/10.1177%2F030631270 5050831.

Prasad, Amit. 2007. "The (Amorphous) Anatomy of an Invention: The Case of Magnetic Resonance Imaging." *Social Studies of Science* 43 (4): 533–60. https://doi.org/10.1177/0306312706075334.

Prasad, Amit. 2008. "Science in Motion: What Postcolonial Science Studies Can Offer." Electronic Journal of Communication Information and Innovation in Health (RECIIS) 2 (2): 35–47. https://doi.org/10.3395/reciis.v2i2.187en.

Prasad, Amit. 2014. *Imperial Technoscience: Transnational Histories of MRI in the United States, Britain, and India*. Cambridge, MA: MIT Press.

Public Accounts Committee. 2005. *Twelfth Report (2004–2005)*. New Delhi: Lok Sabha Secretariat.

Qadeer, Imrana. 2013. "Universal Health Care: The Trojan Horse of Neoliberal Policies." *Social Change* 43 (2): 149–64. https://doi.org/10.1177/0049085713 493037.

Qadeer, Imrana, and Sunita Reddy. 2006. "Scientist Medical Care in the Shadow of Public Private Partnership." *Social Scientist* 34 (9/10): 4–20. https://www.jstor.org/stable/27644167.

Rabinow, Paul. 1996. "Artificiality and Enlightenment: From Sociobiology to Biosociality." In *Essays on the Anthropology of Reason*, edited by Paul Rabinow, 91–111. Princeton, NJ: Princeton University Press.

Ragoné, Helena. 1994. *Surrogate Motherhood: Conception in the Heart*. Boulder, CO: Westview.

Ragoné, Helena. 1996. "Chasing the Blood Tie: Surrogate Mothers, Adoptive Mothers and Fathers." *American Ethnologist* 23 (2): 352–65. https://doi.org/10.1525/ae.1996.23.2.02a00090.

Rahman, Maseeh. 2014. "Genetic Science Existed in Ancient Times: Modi." *The Hindu*, October 30, 2014.

Raina, Dhruv. 1996. "Reconfiguring the Centre: The Structure of Scientific Exchanges between Colonial India and Europe." *Minerva* 34:161–76. https://doi.org/10.1007/BF00122899.

Raina, Dhruv. 2003. *Images and Contexts: The Historiography of Science and Modernity in India*. Delhi: Oxford University Press.

Raj, Kapil. 2010. "Introduction: Circulation and Locality in Early Modern Science." *British Journal for the History of Science* 43:513–17. https://doi.org/10.1017/S0007087410001238.

Raj, Kapil. 2013. "Beyond Postcolonialism . . . and Postpositivism: Circulation and the Global History of Science." *Isis* 104 (2): 337–47. https://doi.org/10.1086/670951.

Rao, Mohan. 2004. *From Population Control to Reproductive Health: Malthusian Arithmetic*. New Delhi: Sage Publications.

Rapp, Rayna. 1999. *Testing Women, Testing the Fetus: The Social Impact of Amniocentesis in America*. New York: Routledge.

Ratzinger, Joseph Card., and Alberto Bovone. 1987. "Congregation for the Doctrine of the Faith: Instruction on the Respect for Human Life in Its Origin and on the Dignity of the Procreation; Replies to Certain Questions of the Day." *Linacre Quarterly* 54 (2): 24–49. https://doi.org/10.1080/00243639.1987.11877891.

Reddy, Sunita, and Tulsi Patel. 2015. "'There Are Many Eggs in My Body': Medical Markets and Commodified Bodies in India." *Global Bioethics* 26 (3–4): 218–31. https://doi.org/10.1080/11287462.2015.1112625.

Rees, Tobias. 2018. *After Ethnos*. Durham, NC: Duke University Press.

Rheinberger, Hans-Jörg. 1994. "Experimental Systems: Historiality, Narration, and Deconstruction." *Science in Context* 7:65–81.

Roberts, Elizabeth F. S. 2007. "Extra Embryos: The Ethics of Cryopreservation in Ecuador and Elsewhere." *American Ethnologist* 34 (1): 181–99. https://doi.org/10.1525/ae.2007.34.1.181.

Roberts, Elizabeth F. S. 2012. *God's Laboratory: Assisted Reproduction in the Andes*. Berkeley: University of California Press.

Rosaldo, Renato. 1989. *Culture and Truth: The Remaking of Social Analysis*. Boston: Beacon.

Ruckenstein, Minna, and Natasha Dow Schüll. 2017. "The Datafication of Health." *Annual Review of Anthropology* 46:261–78. https://doi.org/10.1146/annurev-anthro-102116-041244.

Rudrappa, Sharmila. 2015. *Discounted Life: The Price of Global Surrogacy in India*. New York: NYU Press.

Sahlins, Marshall. 1999. "What Is Anthropological Enlightenment? Some Lessons of the Twentieth Century." *Annual Review of Anthropology* 28:i–xxiii. https://doi.org/10.1146/annurev.anthro.28.1.0.

Sahlins, Marshall. 2013. *What Kinship Is—and Is Not*. Chicago: University of Chicago Press.

Sama Resource Group for Women and Health. 2010. *Constructing Conceptions: The Mapping of Assisted Reproductive Technologies in India*. New Delhi. http://www.samawomenshealth.in/constructing-conceptions/.

Sanabria, Emilia. 2016. *Plastic Bodies: Sex Hormones and Menstrual Suppression in Brazil*. Durham, NC: Duke University Press.

Saravanan, Sheela. 2010. "Transnational Surrogacy and Objectification of Gestational Mothers." *Economic and Political Weekly* 45 (16):26–29. https://www.epw.in/journal/2010/16/commentary/transnational-surrogacy-and-objectification-gestational-mothers.html.

Saravanan, Sheela. 2018. *A Transnational Feminist View of Surrogacy Biomarkets in India*. Singapore: Springer.

Sarojini Nadimpally, Vrinda Marwah, and Anjali Shenoi. 2011. "Globalisation of Birth Markets: A Case Study of Assisted Reproductive Technologies in India." *Globalization and Health* 7 (27): 1–9. https://doi.org/10.1186/1744-8603-7-27.

Schneider, David M. 1980. *American Kinship: A Cultural Account*. Chicago: University of Chicago Press.

Sengoopta, Chandak. 2006. *The Most Secret Quintessence of Life: Sex, Glands, and Hormones, 1850–1950*. Chicago: University of Chicago Press.

Sengupta, Amit, and Samiran Nundy. 2005. "The Private Health Sector in India Is Burgeoning, but at the Cost of Public Health Care." *BMJ* 331:1157–58. https://doi.org/10.1136/bmj.331.7526.1157.

Sengupta, Amit, and Vandana Prasad. 2011. "Developing a Truly Universal Indian Health System: The Problem of Replacing 'Health for All' with 'Universal Access to Health Care.'" *Social Medicine* 6 (2): 69–72. https://www.socialmedicine.info/index.php/socialmedicine/article/view/587.

Serres, Michel. 1998. *Conversations on Science, Culture, and Time: Michel Serres with Bruno Latour*. Translated by Roxanne Lapidus. Ann Arbor: University of Michigan Press.

Shapin, Steven. 1988. "The House of Experiment in Seventeenth-Century England." *Isis* 79 (3): 373–404. https://www.jstor.org/stable/234672.

Shapiro, Nicholas, and Eben Kirksey. 2017. "Chemo-Ethnography: An Introduction." *Cultural Anthropology* 32 (4): 481–93. https://doi.org/10.14506/ca32.4.01.

Sharp, Lesley A. 2001. "Commodified Kin: Death, Mourning, and Competing Claims on the Bodies of Organ Donors in the United States." *American Anthropologist* 103 (1): 112–33. https://doi.org/10.1525/aa.2001.103.1.112.

Simpson, Bob. 2004a. "Gays, Paternity, and Polyandry: Making Sense of New Family Forms in Contemporary Sri Lanka." In *South Asian Masculinities: Context of Change, Sites of Continuity*, edited by Radhika Chopra, Caroline Osella, and Filippo Osella, 160–74. New Delhi: Women Unlimited.

Simpson, Bob. 2004b. "Impossible Gifts: Bodies, Buddhism and Bioethics in Contemporary Sri Lanka." *Journal of the Royal Anthropological Institute* 10 (4): 839–59. https://doi.org/10.1111/j.1467-9655.2004.00214.x.

Simpson, Bob. 2011. "Blood Rhetorics: Donor Campaigns and Their Publics in Contemporary Sri Lanka." *Ethnos* 76 (2): 254–75. https://doi.org/10.1080/00141844.2010.546868.

Simpson, Bob. 2013. "Managing Potential in Assisted Reproductive Technologies: Reflections on Gifts, Kinship, and the Process of Vernacularization." *Current Anthropology* 54 (S7): S87–S96. https://doi.org/10.1086/670173.

Singh, Holly Donahue. 2017. "Fertility Control: Reproductive Desires, Kin Work, and Women's Status in Contemporary India." *Medical Anthropology Quarterly* 31 (1): 23–39. https://doi.org/10.1111/maq.12312.

Spriggs, Merle. 2003. "IVF Mixup: White Couple Have Black Babies." *Journal of Medical Ethics* 29 (2): 65. http://dx.doi.org/10.1136/jme.29.2.65.

Srinivasan, Vasanthi, and Rajesh Chandwani. 2014. "HRM Innovations in Rapid Growth Contexts: The Healthcare Sector in India." *International Journal of Human Resource Management* 25 (10): 1505–25. https://doi.org/10.1080/09585192.2013.870308.

Star, Susan Leigh. 2002. "Infrastructure and Ethnographic Practice: Working on the Fringes." *Scandinavian Journal of Information Systems* 14 (2): 107–22. http://aisel.aisnet.org/sjis/vol14/iss2/6.

Statesman, The. 1980. "Scheme to Extract Hormone from Urine." January 22, 1980.

Stengers, Isabelle. 2003. "The Doctor and the Charlatan." *Cultural Studies Review* 9 (2): 11–36. https://doi.org/10.5130/csr.v9i2.3561.

Strathern, Marilyn. 1992. *After Nature: English Kinship in the Late Twentieth Century*. Cambridge: Cambridge University Press.

Strathern, Marilyn. 1995. *The Relation: Issues in Complexity and Scale*. Cambridge: Prickly Pear.

Strathern, Marilyn. 1999. "Refusing Information." In *Property, Substance, and Effect: Anthropological Essays on Persons and Things*, edited by Marilyn Strathern, 64–88. London: Athlone.

Street, Alice. 2014. *Biomedicine in an Unstable Place: Infrastructure and Personhood in a Papua New Guinean Hospital*. Durham, NC: Duke University Press.

Street, Alice, and Simon Coleman. 2012. "Introduction: Real and Imagined Spaces." *Space and Culture* 15 (1): 4–17. https://doi.org/10.1177%2F1206331211421852.

Sturken, Marita, and Lisa Cartwright. 2009. *Practices of Looking: An Introduction to Visual Culture*. Oxford: Oxford University Press.

Sujatha, V. 2014. *Sociology of Health and Medicine: New Perspectives*. Delhi: Oxford University Press.

Sunder Rajan, Kaushik. 2006. *Biocapital: The Constitution of Postgenomic Life*. Durham, NC: Duke University Press.

Sunder Rajan, Kaushik. 2012. "Introduction: The Capitalization of Life and the Liveliness of Capital." In *Lively Capital: Biotechnologies, Ethics, and Governance in Global Markets*, edited by Kaushik Sunder Rajan, 1–41. Durham, NC: Duke University Press.

Sur, Sayantani. 2017. "Bodies in Poverty: Family Planning and Poverty Removal in India." *Economic and Political Weekly* 52 (40): 48–56. https://www.epw.in/journal/2017/40/special-articles/bodies-poverty.html.

Tanderup, Malene, Sunita Reddy, Tulsi Patel, and Birgitte Bruun Nielsen. 2015. "Reproductive Ethics in Commercial Surrogacy: Decision-Making in IVF Clinics in New Delhi, India." *Bioethical Inquiry* 12:491–501. https://doi.org/10.1007/s11673-015-9642-8.

Tarlo, Emma. 2003. *Unsettling Memories: Narratives of the Emergency in Delhi*. Berkeley: University of California Press.

Tausk, Marius. 1984. *Organon: The Story of an Unusual Pharmaceutical Enterprise*. Oss, Netherlands: Akzo Pharma.

Thomas, George, and Suneeta Krishnan. 2010. "Effective Public-Private Partnership in Healthcare: Apollo as a Cautionary Tale." *Indian Journal of Medical Ethics* 7 (1): 2–4. https://doi.org/10.20529/IJME.2010.001.

Thompson, Charis. 2005. *Making Parents: The Ontological Choreography of Reproductive Technologies*. Cambridge, MA: MIT Press.

Tikku, Aloke. 2013. "ICMR Has Not Delayed Surrogacy Law: RS Sharma." *Hindustan Times*, November 12, 2013.

Traweek, Sharon. 1992. "Big Science and Colonialist Discourse: Building High-Energy Physics in Japan." In *Big Science: The Growth of Large Scale Research*, edited by Peter Galison and Bruce William Hevly, 100–128. Stanford, CA: Stanford University Press.

Trommelen, Jeroen. 2013. "Zwangere vrouwen misleid door farmaceutisch bedrijf." *De Volkskrant*, May 27, 2013.

Tsing, Anna. 2013. "Sorting Out Commodities: How Capitalist Value Is Made through Gifts." *HAU: Journal of Ethnographic Theory* 3 (1): 21–43. https://doi.org/10.14318/hau3.1.003.

Tsing, Anna. 2015. *The Mushroom at the End of the World: On the Possibility of Life in Capitalist Ruins*. Princeton, NJ: Princeton University Press.

Turner, Leigh. 2007. "'First World Health Care at Third World Prices': Globalization, Bioethics and Medical Tourism." *BioSocieties* 2 (3): 303–25. https://doi.org/10.1017/S1745855207005765.

United Nations Population Fund. 2014. *Programme of Action Adopted at the International Conference on Population and Development Cairo 5–13 September 1994*. 20th anniversary ed. https://www.unfpa.org/publications/international-conference-population-and-development-programme-action.

Unnithan, Maya. 2010. "Infertility and Assisted Reproductive Technologies (ARTs) in Globalising India: Ethics, Medicalisation and Agency." *Asian Bioethics Review* 2 (1): 3–18. https://muse.jhu.edu/article/416374.

van der Geest, Sjaak, and Kaja Finkler. 2004. "Hospital Ethnography: Introduction." *Social Science and Medicine* 59 (10): 1995–2001. https://doi.org/10.1016/j.socs cimed.2004.03.004.

van de Wiel, Lucy. 2019. "The Datafication of Reproduction: Time-Lapse Embryo Imaging and the Commercialisation of IVF." *Sociology of Health & Illness* 41 (S1): 193–209. https://doi.org/10.1111/1467-9566.12881.

Vatin, François. 2013. "Valuation as Evaluating and Valorizing." *Valuation Studies* 1 (1): 31–50. https://doi.org/10.3384/vs.2001-5992.131131.

Verhoog, J. 1998. *75 Years: Organon; 1923–1998*. Oss, Netherlands: N.V. Organon.

Vertommen, Sigrid. 2017. "From the Pergonal Project to Kadimastem: A Genealogy of Israel's Reproductive-Industrial Complex." *BioSocieties* 12 (2): 282–306. https:// doi.org/10.1057/biosoc.2015.44.

Viveiros de Castro, Eduardo. 2009. "The Gift and the Given: Three Nano-Essays on Kinship and Magic." In *Kinship and Beyond: The Genealogical Model Reconsidered*, edited by Sandra Bamford and James Leach, 237–68. New York: Berghahn Books.

Vora, Kalindi. 2013. "Potential, Risk, and Return in Transnational Indian Gestational Surrogacy." *Current Anthropology* 54 (S7): S97–S106. https://doi.org/10.1086/671018.

Wahlberg, Ayo. 2008. "Reproductive Medicine and the Concept of 'Quality.'" *Clinical Ethics* 3 (4): 189–93. https://doi.org/10.1258/ce.2008.008033.

Wahlberg, Ayo. 2018. *Good Quality: The Routinization of Sperm Banking in China*. Oakland: University of California Press.

Waldby, Catherine. 2019. *The Oocyte Economy: The Changing Meaning of Human Eggs*. Durham, NC: Duke University Press.

Waldby, Catherine, and Robert Mitchell. 2006. *Tissue Economies: Blood, Organs, and Cell Lines in Late Capitalism*. Durham, NC: Duke University Press.

Whittaker, Andrea. 2015. *Thai In Vitro: Gender, Culture and Assisted Reproduction*. New York: Berghahn Books.

Whittaker, Andrea, and Amy Speier. 2010. "'Cycling Overseas': Care, Commodification, and Stratification in Cross-Border Reproductive Travel." *Medical Anthropology* 29 (4): 363–83. https://doi.org/10.1080/01459740.2010.501313.

Widge, Anjali. 2001. "Sociocultural Attitudes towards Infertility and Assisted Reproduction in India." In *Current Practices and Controversies in Assisted Reproduction: Report of a WHO Meeting on "Medical, Ethical and Social Aspects of Assisted Reproduction,"* edited by Effy Vayena, Patrick J. Rowe, and P. David Griffin, 60–74. Geneva: World Health Organization. https://www.who.int/repro ductivehealth/publications/infertility/9241590300/en/.

Widge, Anjali. 2005. "Seeking Conception: Experiences of Urban Indian Women with In Vitro Fertilization." *Patient Education and Counseling* 59 (3): 226–33. https:// doi.org/10.1016/j.pec.2005.07.014.

Widge, Anjali, and John Cleland. 2009. "Assisted Reproductive Technologies in India: The Views of Practitioners." *Human Fertility* 12 (3): 144–52. https://doi. org/10.1080/14647270903212156.

Wilson, Kristin J. 2014. *Not Trying: Infertility, Childlessness, and Ambivalence*. Nashville: Vanderbilt University Press.

Wind, Gitte. 2008. "Negotiated Interactive Observation: Doing Fieldwork in Hospital Settings." *Anthropology and Medicine* 15 (2): 79–89. https://doi.org/10.1080/13648 470802127098.

World Health Organization (Department of Reproductive Health and Research). 2010. *WHO Laboratory Manual for the Examination and Processing of Human Semen*. 5th ed. https://www.who.int/reproductivehealth/publications/infertility/97892 41547789/en/.

Zegers-Hochschild, Fernando, G. David Adamson, Jacques de Mouzon, Osamu Ishihara, Ragaa Mansour, Karl Nygren, Elisabeth Sullivan, and Sheryl Vanderpoel. 2009. "International Committee for Monitoring Assisted Reproductive Technology (ICMART) and the World Health Organization (WHO) Revised Glossary of ART Terminology." *Fertility and Sterility* 92 (5): 1520–24. https://doi.org/10.1016/j.fertn stert.2009.09.009.

Zimmermann, Francis. 2014. "Medical Individualism and the Dividual Person." In *Asymmetrical Conversations: Contestations, Circumventions, and the Blurring of Therapeutic Boundaries*, edited by Harish Naraindas, Johannes Quack, and William S. Sax, 85–117. New York: Berghahn Books.

Index

Page numbers in italics refer to figures.

abortion, 51, 130, 134, 144n20
adoption, 79, 81, 92, 96, 106, 110–11, 147n3
adulteration, 34–35, 104
adultery, 105
Agarwal family, 44, 46, 50–51
ampoules, 24, 30–31, 34. *See also* hCG;
    Pregnyl
Anand Kumar, T. C., 46–47, 49, 51, 55, 58, 63,
    145n8
anxieties: about mix-ups and boundary
    crossings, 20, 101–4, 112–13, 116–17;
    about possible abnormalities, 44–45, 51;
    prevalence of, 139
archival research, 15
Aspen Pharma, 143n8
assisted reproductive technologies, 1–6.
    See also global reproductive
    medicine; ICSI; infertility management;
    IUI; IVF
Assisted Reproductive Technology (Regulation)
    Bill (2020), 14, 56, 108, 111, 113, 116, 122,
    140, 145n6, 148n11

Bengal Obstetrics and Gynaecological Society,
    45, 53
Bhattacharya, Saroj Kanti, 42
Bhore Committee, 66, 145n5(chap.3)
bioeconomies, 8, 12, 24
biological substances, 1, 5–10; relational
    constitution of, 9–10, 139; relational
    potential, 7–9, 103–5; transnational
    flows of, 6–7, 18–19, 22–37, 137, 141n12.
    See also bodies; egg cells; embryos;
    gametes; hCG; reproductive substances;
    semen; sperm; urine
biosociality, 115
birth control, 11
bodies: chronological and gynecological age
    of, 83; corporeal generosity, 29–31; mal-
    leability and resistance, 100; productivity,
    29–31, 85–86, 100, 147n10; relations and,
    9–10; response of, 85–87; somatic activity,

100; somatic rhythms, 84–88, 100; unpre-
    dictability of, 86, 100. *See also* biological
    substances
Bose, Satyendra Nath, 53
boundary transgressions, 20, 101–4, 112–13,
    115–17
Bourn Hall Clinic, UK, 13, 63
bricolage, 56
Brown, Louise, 42, 46, 63

capitalism, 20, 24, 116, 138
caste, 7–8, 20, 28, 101–4, 110–11, 115–17
Catholic Church, 129, 143n7
Chakraborty, Baidyanath, 1–3, 53–55, 60–61,
    145n1
charitable hospitals, 65–66, 69, 71, 74. *See also*
    hospitals
Chhetri, Mani, 43
childbearing, 79, 106, 134, 147n11,
    148n4(chap. 5). *See also* IVF babies
classed relations, 24; donor gametes and, 108,
    115–16; IVF research and, 149n12; urine
    collection programs and, 28, 34–36.
    See also middle-class patients; working-
    class patients
clinical practice, 20, 76–100, 139–40; bodily
    rhythms and, 84–88, 100; division of med-
    ical labor, 67; improvised interventions,
    60–64, 74; mundane, 78, 139; objects of,
    20 (*see also* bodies; embryos; gametes).
    See also doctors; embryologists; IVF
colonialism, 8–9, 13, 36, 54
commercial donors, 107–9, 116–17, 148n7.
    See also donor gametes
conception, natural, 96–97, 147n15
contraceptive pill, 26, 33, 84, 144n13
corporate hospitals, 60, 69–71, 75,
    146n7(chap. 3). *See also* hospitals
corporeal matter, 6–7, 141n12. *See also*
    biological substances; bodies
costs: of corporate hospitals, 146n7(chap. 3);
    high-cost hospitals, 9, 72, 75, 115, 140; of

Lightning Source UK Ltd.
Milton Keynes UK
UKHW010657101121
393711UK00003B/145